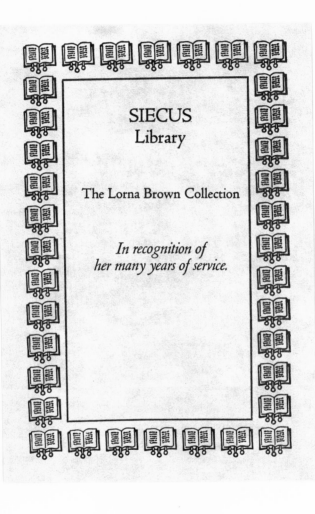

THE SEX HANDBOOK

Information and Help for Minors

THE SEX HANDBOOK

INFORMATION AND HELP FOR MINORS

Heidi Handman and Peter Brennan

Illustrated by Emmett McConnell

FOUNDED 1838
GPPS

G. P. PUTNAM'S SONS, New York

1974

Published simultaneously in Canada
by Longman Canada Limited, Toronto.

SBN: 399-11258-8
Library of Congress Catalog Card Number: 73-87191

Printed in the United States of America

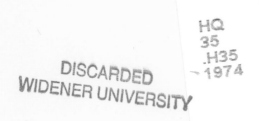

About This Book

This book is written for men and women under 18. It's designed to give you all the information you need to enjoy sex and take care of yourself.

This book doesn't say much about love. That's not because emotions aren't important—it's because you already know your own feelings better than anybody else.

This book concentrates on practical information that's hard to get—information about your body, about having sex, about getting birth control and other kinds of help on your own.

CONTENTS

THE SEX HANDBOOK
Information and Help for Minors

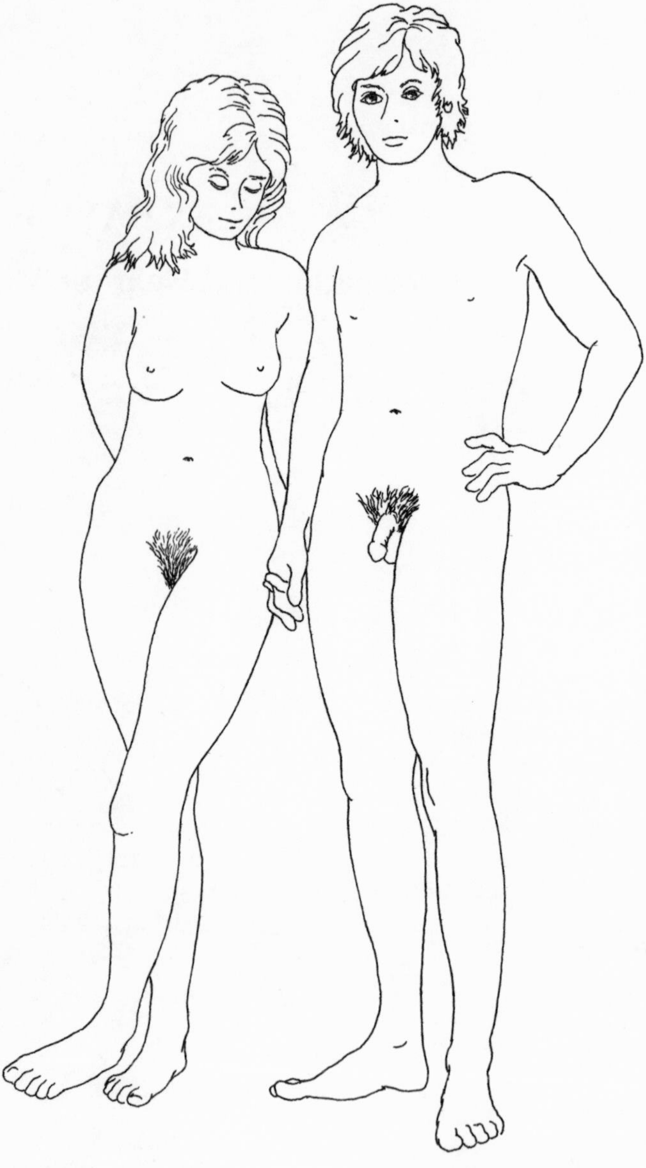

1

SEX AND FREEDOM

Sex is a natural appetite. It comes from your body like hunger or thirst or the need to sleep. And when your body is ready to have sex, you can feel it.

Your body becomes sexually mature during puberty. That means you're not only capable of having children but also of experiencing a wide range of sexual pleasures and passions.

But as long as you're under eighteen, having any kind of sex can be a hassle. Parents, schools, churches, and even the government try to make it as difficult as possible to enjoy your own body.

Parents pretend sex doesn't exist.

Schools won't teach you what you need to know.

Churches preach that sex is immoral.

And the government makes it illegal for minors to have sex—or even see it on a movie screen.

In school they talk about your body like it's some kind of factory. It's all ovaries and spermatozoa. They may tell you how your sex organs can produce children, but they never mention how your entire body can be handled to produce pleasure.

Sex is a lot more than just reproduction.

Sex is digging your own body because it feels good.

Sex is giving pleasure to somebody you like.

Sex is a way of communicating with your body. It involves tenderness and intimacy and lots of strong feelings.

And while sex is a natural instinct, nobody is born with any special knowledge or talent. We all have to learn how to be good at sex, just like we have to learn everything else.

There's a certain amount of experimentation involved in learning about sex. And despite everything adults would like you to believe, having sex won't hurt you.

If you're old enough to want sex, you're old enough to have it.

SEX AND SOCIETY

We live in a sexually repressive society. And people under eighteen are the major victims of this repression.

For hundreds of years our society has believed that sex is some kind of sin. And every kind of sex outside of marriage has been forbidden—especially for people under eighteen.

In primitive cultures men and women are allowed to have sex as soon as they're ready. In our so-called civilized society we're told to wait and wait long after our bodies have become hungry.

In every other way we're encouraged to grow and develop as soon as possible. Parents are so proud when their kids learn to walk and talk and read—but horrified when they learn to fuck.

Sex is the one thing we're not supposed to know anything about or be good at. And in order to prevent young people from having sex, society uses a combination of censorship, silence, and outright prohibition.

All of this creates problems. For one thing it means that sex has to be a secret activity. Everything from masturbating to balling has to be hidden—especially from parents.

It's also difficult to get any real information about sex. Most people have to learn about sex from their friends. Sometimes friends know what they're talking about; sometimes they don't. There are still lots of myths and misunderstandings about sex that get passed around.

As a result of society's attitude, minors suffer from more problems like accidental pregnancy and venereal disease than any other age group. And while these are real problems, they're both completely unnecessary.

Safe, reliable birth control already exists, and the danger of VD can be greatly reduced with a little information. But parents never mention these subjects, and in many places it's illegal to teach them in the classroom. In addition, the law in many states makes it difficult for minors to get birth control and medical care on their own.

If you're under eighteen, society tries to put all kinds of obstacles in the way of your sexual freedom. But you can get around a lot of those obstacles if you want to. All you need is the right information and a little help.

SEX AND MORALITY

It's impossible to talk about sex in this society without always hearing about morality.

All you have to do is mention sex, and most middle-aged people start to sound as pious as Billy Graham. They don't seem half as upset about war or poverty as they do about young people enjoying their bodies.

But people who go around condemning the "sexual immorality of youth" are either hypocrites or they're terribly frightened by sex. And if they haven't had much sexual pleasure in their own lives, they don't want other people to get what they missed.

Sex is a natural, healthy part of life, and our morals about sex should be the same as they are for everything else. Our bodies are never immoral, and neither is sexual pleasure. But there can be something wrong with the way we treat other people.

For example, forcing somebody to do what they don't want is wrong.

Exploiting somebody's feelings is wrong.

Being dishonest with your sexual partner is wrong.

If you say you love somebody when all you really want is to get laid, then you're fucking around with your partner's emotions. If you sleep with somebody when you've got VD, then you're fucking around with your partner's body.

In any of these things it's not the sex that is wrong. It's hurting or cheating or deceiving another person.

As long as two people are honest with each other, and they know where each other's heads are at, then sex is never immoral. And anything two people do together that gives them both pleasure is good.

SEX IS YOUR OWN BUSINESS

Sex is a personal thing.

Nobody can tell you when you should have sex or why you should have sex. Your body belongs to you, and sex is your own decision.

Your body is ready to have sex as soon as you reach puberty. But sex also involves your emotions. Whether or not you want to have sex—any kind of sex—depends on how you feel.

There are many reasons for having sex, and most people have different feelings at different times.

There's sex for the physical pleasure. After all, sex feels good and it's fun. Two people who are attracted to each other can have enjoyable sex—with or without any other kind of relationship.

There's sex to express your feelings. Making it with somebody you really care about is a way of getting closer together—emotionally as well as physically.

There's sex for curiosity. Lots of people have sex just for the experience. Other people have sex to find out something about themselves—or their partner.

Sex can be whatever you want. It can be a casual thing or a serious way of showing love. There's no one reason for enjoying your own body.

And there's no correct age for everybody to start having sex either.

Some people are eager to have sex as soon as they can. Other people want to wait for the right relationship. We're all different; our personalities are unique. And we don't have to be like anybody else.

Of course it's hard to ignore other people completely. Parents can make you feel guilty if you have sex; friends can make you feel uptight if you don't. But other people can't know what's right for you.

Everybody has different sexual feelings. Everybody has different sexual needs. And the important thing is to follow your own instincts.

Sexual freedom doesn't mean you have to fuck everybody you meet. It means being free to do what you want when you want. Free to say yes and free to say no.

Freedom involves your head as well as your body.

2

SEX ORGANS

You don't have to know much about your body to have sex. You don't have to know much about your partner's body. But the more you do know, the more you can enjoy sex. Understanding what's happening with your own body and your partner's makes sex better and a lot more meaningful.

From the outside, male and female bodies may look very different—especially the sex organs. But men and women have a lot more in common than most people realize. We're both made out of the same mold.

During the first few months of life in the womb, it's almost impossible to tell the difference between males and females. We both look the same. Only gradually do certain physical changes make us into separate sexes.

But almost every sexual organ in one sex has its counterpart in the other sex.

The male penis and the female clitoris both grow in the same place and develop out of the same kind of skin. The sensitive skin that forms the lips of the female vagina is the same skin that forms the scrotum in the male.

And both sexes have a similar pair of glands that control our sexual development. In the female these glands are the ovaries, which are inside the abdomen. The male glands are testicles, and they also develop in the abdomen. But right before birth the testicles drop down into the scrotum.

We may look different, and our sex organs may work differently, but both male and female are made out of very similar stuff. And if we understand our own body—how it works, how it feels, how it responds—it should help us understand our partner's body. And that's what sex is all about.

THE FEMALE GENITALS

The best way for a woman to learn about her sexual anatomy is to hold a mirror between her legs and take a good, long look at her own genitals.

All the medical diagrams that you've seen will make a lot more sense when you compare them to your own sexual parts. And you've got to know what your own sex organs look like before you can really understand how they function.

A woman's genitals undergo a series of physical reactions during sex. The shape, the size, and even the color of the genitals change when a woman is sexually excited. If you know what to expect, it's easy to recognize these changes in your own body.

The Vulva

The whole area between a woman's legs is called the vulva. It includes all the external parts of the genitals: the outer and inner lips, the clitoris, the urethra, and the opening of the vagina.

The outer lips are the two thick folds of skin that are covered with hair. Technically they're called the labia majora. Most of the time these lips lie close together, protecting the more delicate skin underneath. But when your body becomes sexually excited,

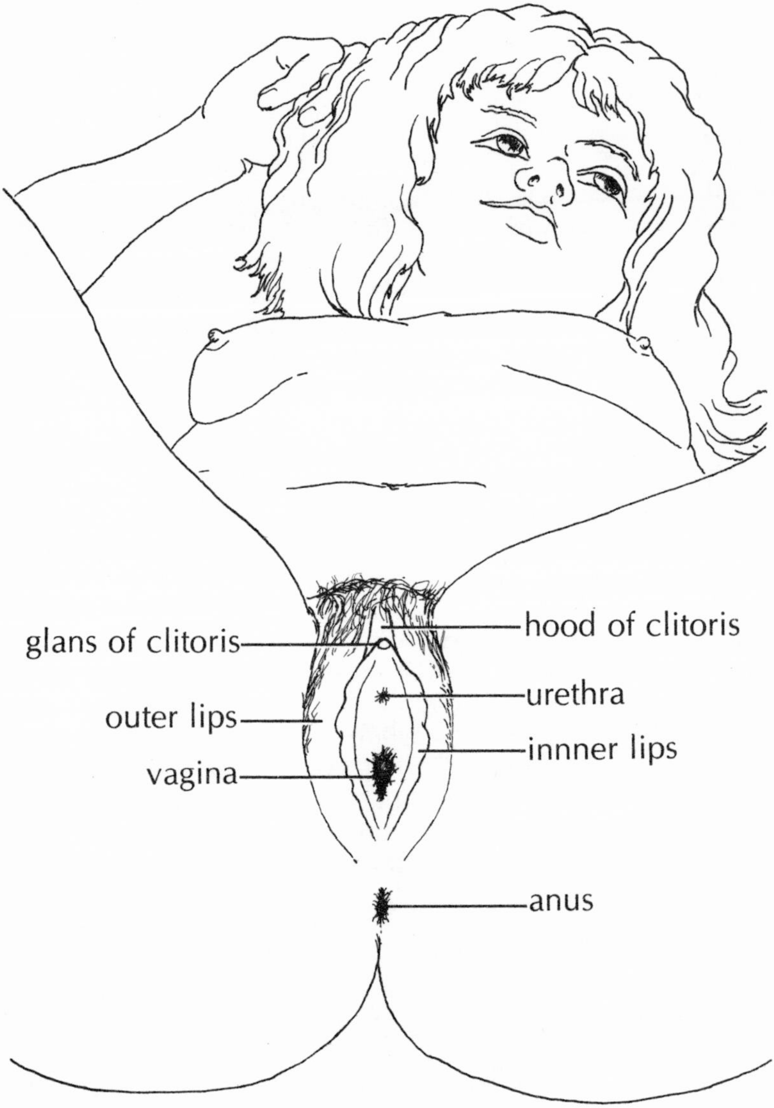

THE VULVA: a woman's external sexual parts

blood fills the gential area and makes the outer lips swell and spread apart.

When the outer lips are separated, you can see the inner lips, called labia minora. They're darker, thinner, and more slippery than the outer lips, with ruffled edges like a rooster's comb.

Like the outer lips, the inner lips also swell and spread apart when you're sexually excited. But they're much more sensitive to touch. You can test that yourself by stroking them both and seeing how differently they feel. Because of their sensitivity, the inner lips are an important source of sexual pleasure for a woman.

The clitoris is the most sensitive part of a woman's sexual anatomy. This small organ, shaped like an upside-down ice cream cone, starts at the top of the vulva where the outer lips come together.

The clitoris is made up of several parts. The large cone-shaped part is actually a hood. Underneath this hood of skin is the shaft of the clitoris. But only the tiny, round end of it, called the glans, is visible. If you examine your clitoris, you may notice the glans peeking out from under the hood, or you may have to pull back the hood in order to see the glans emerge.

When a woman is sexually excited, she feels the pleasure in her clitoris. Of course the whole vulva—and the whole body—feels pleasure during sex, but strong sexual sensations are concentrated in the clitoris. And this is true even if the clitoris hasn't been touched. If you're turned on by having your breasts stroked or by a penis moving in and out of your vagina or even by thinking about sex, the erotic feelings are focused in the clitoris.

Like the rest of a woman's sexual anatomy, the clitoris goes through physical changes during sexual excitement. It gets bigger and harder as it fills with blood, and the tiny glans pokes out further from its hood. Right before a woman has an orgasm, the glans of the clitoris pulls back under the hood and stays there until orgasm is over.

Between the clitoris and the vagina is the small hole through which a woman urinates. This is the opening to the urethra, a tube which leads to the bladder. The urethral opening is very sensitive to touch. Some women find it erotic to stimulate the urethra, but others find it unpleasant or downright painful. In either case, it's a functional part of the genital anatomy and doesn't play a big role in sex one way or the other.

The Vagina

The opening of a woman's vagina can be seen by pulling apart the inner lips. This hole is much bigger than the urethra, and it's shaped like a funnel. The wide end is the smooth, sensitive, external skin, and the narrow end is a hard ring of muscle that you can feel by putting a finger an inch or two inside the hole.

A woman who has never had intercourse, however, may find the entrance to her vagina blocked by a thin sheet of skin. This is called the hymen, or cherry. The hymen is elastic tissue that has a few perforations in it to allow the menstrual flow to leave the body.

Breaking the hymen is what causes pain and bleeding in some women when they get laid for the first time. But a woman can be born without a hymen, and many women stretch or break their hymen long before they get around to having intercourse.

The inside of the vagina is a tube that connects the internal reproductive organs with the outside world. The walls of the vagina lie against each other, collapsed like an empty balloon.

The vagina is very elastic, and it expands to the size of whatever is inside it. If you insert a tampon, the vagina expands to the size of the tampon. If a penis is inserted into the vagina, it expands to the size of the penis. And it can become as big as the baby that passes through it during childbirth.

If you put your finger inside the vagina, you can feel the rippled muscles of the outer third and the smoother texture of the deeper recesses of the vagina. When a woman gets sexually excited, the outer muscles become tense, and the inner walls separate from each other. The entire vagina becomes longer and wider.

The vagina also reacts to sexual excitement in other ways.

A woman may notice that her vagina feels very wet when she's aroused. The vaginal walls secrete a fluid that serves as a lubricant and makes it easier for a penis to enter.

And when a woman has an orgasm, the ring of muscles inside the vagina contracts in a series of spasms. You can feel these contractions if you keep a finger inside the vagina when you come.

There are lots of misconceptions about the vagina. Probably the biggest mistake that people make is thinking that the inside of the vagina is the center of a woman's sexual feelings. While the outer third of the vagina is very sensitive to touch, the deeper recesses are almost totally insensitive. You can feel pressure inside the vagina, but not much else. There are very few nerve endings inside it, so there can't possibly be much feeling there. Sexual activity may center in the vagina, but sexual pleasure is centered in the clitoris.

Some people worry about the size of the vagina. Everybody's heard stories about the girl whose cunt was so big that a cock would just flop around inside it or the girl whose vagina was so small she couldn't fuck at all. These stories are bullshit. All vaginas are just about the same size, and they expand and contract to conform to the size of a man's penis.

Many people also believe that a woman's vagina ejaculates during orgasm just like a man's penis. This is absolutely untrue. The vagina gets wet when it lubricates during sexual excitement, but there is no ejaculation when a woman comes.

The Breasts

A woman's breasts are probably the most obvious part of her sexual anatomy. They can start to develop when a girl is only ten years old, or they may not reach their full size until the age of eighteen.

Many women notice that their breasts change in size and sensitivity during the course of a month. For example, they may get bigger and become especially tender right before your period. The breasts react to the changing level of sex hormones in a woman's body, which varies according to her menstrual cycle.

The nipples and the dark circle of skin surrounding them are the most sensitive parts of the breasts. They respond to touch, to sexual stimulation, and even to temperature. You'll notice they crinkle up if you step out of a hot bath into the cold air.

The breasts also go through changes during sexual excitement —just like the genitals. They swell and increase in size. In fact, the breasts can increase by as much as a quarter of their usual size. The nipples become erect, and the dark skin around them contracts into tight ridges. These changes happen even if the breasts haven't been directly touched.

Breast size is often confused with a woman's sexuality. People seem to think that big tits make for a more sexual woman. But in reality size has absolutely nothing to do with the sensitivity of a woman's breasts.

Most women, in fact, have two slightly different-sized breasts. No one's body is perfectly symmetrical. It's normal to have one breast that's a little larger than the other, just like it's normal to have one foot that's a little larger than the other.

And small breasts are just as sexually responsive as big ones. How much a woman likes sex really depends on where her head is at, not on the size or shape of her tits.

The Anus

The anus is one part of the body that many people don't associate with sex. But it is part of your sexual anatomy. Like the vagina, it's sensitive at the opening but not deep inside. When a woman has an orgasm, the anus sometimes contracts in spasms like the vagina. It's often pleasant to have the anus touched during sex. Try it. If you like it, then it's just one more way to enhance sexual pleasure.

THE MALE GENITALS

When you look at a man's body, the external sex organs, the penis and the testicles, are rather hard to miss. Most men are as familiar with every wrinkle and fold in their genitals as they are with their hands. Exploring your own sex organs is natural and unavoidable for most men.

The Penis

The penis is probably the most elastic organ in the male body. One minute it's soft and crinkled up, the next minute it's swollen and hard. Almost any kind of sexual stimulation makes the cock erect. Looking at a woman's body, being touched or kissed—just thinking about sex can cause an erection.

Sometimes it seems like you walk around with an erection half your life. You wake up in the morning and your cock is liable to be hard, you get an erection sitting in school, just having to take a piss makes your cock stand up.

The penis is a long tube of spongelike erectile tissue. Normally blood circulates in and out of the penis at the same rate. But at the first sign of sexual excitement, a ring of muscles around the base of the penis contracts and slows down the flow of blood out of the organ. The spongy tissues inside the penis fill up with blood, making it expand and stiffen.

You can test this action yourself by squeezing tight around the base of the penis—right where it meets the body. By cutting off the flow of blood out of the cock you can make an erect penis even fuller and larger.

The most sensitive part of the penis is the head. It's made of smooth, delicate tissue filled with thousands of nerve endings similar to the glans of a woman's clitoris. During masturbation or intercourse the head of the penis gets direct stimulation.

The hole in the top of the penis is the opening to a tube called the urethra, which runs through the center of the penis. At the base of the cock the urethra branches out into two parts—one tube goes to the bladder, one tube goes to the testicles. The urine from a man's bladder and the semen from his reproductive organs pass through the urethra and out the end of the penis.

But you can't piss and come at the same time. A switch at the base of the penis regulates which of the tubes is open. Normally the tube to the bladder is open. But when you get sexually excited, a valve closes off that tube and opens up the tube to the testicles. It can't be open both ways at the same time. In fact, it's impossible to piss when you have an erection even if you want to—you have to wait for the penis to go soft again.

When an erection goes down, the muscles at the base of the penis relax and let the blood flow back into the rest of the body.

All of these physical functions are involuntary—they're triggered automatically by the brain. Which is just as well, because when you get sexually excited, nobody wants to think about blood vessels and valves and erectile tissue.

PENIS SIZE

Most men, unless they're born with cocks that hang down to their knees, worry about whether their penis is big enough. The fact is, almost all men have the same size sexual organs. Cock size can vary a lot when the penis is soft—expanding and contracting continually throughout the day—but at full erection most cocks measure five to six inches long. Undoubtedly there are some people with larger organs, just like there are some people who stand close to seven feet tall—but they're the exception, not the average.

And the size of the cock, contrary to popular myths, has nothing to do with sexual potency. A penis has to be only as long as a finger to give a woman sexual pleasure, since the vagina expands and contracts to grip whatever is inserted into it. And there's absolutely no relation between cock size and the power of your own orgasm.

CIRCUMCISION

The most common difference in male genitals is not their size but whether or not the penis is circumcised.

All males are born with a hood of skin—the foreskin—covering the head of the penis. Circumcision is the surgical removal of this foreskin. It's a simple operation that is usually performed within several weeks after birth.

Circumcision began as a primitive religious ritual several thousand years ago. But the custom has spread to many religions and cultures. Today circumcision of infant males is common in this country because it's believed that the penis is easier to keep clean without the foreskin. Also, many people prefer the way the penis looks when it's been circumcised.

Men who have been circumcised inevitably think it's better to have the foreskin removed. Men who haven't been circumcised claim that losing the foreskin decreases the sensitivity of the penis and that it's better to leave the organ in its natural state. But medical studies like those conducted by Masters and Johnson, a famous team of sex researchers, show that there is no difference between a circumcised and uncircumcised penis in sexual sensitivity. Foreskin or no foreskin, fucking feels the same—to both the male and his female partner.

When the uncircumcised penis is soft, the head is usually hidden under the foreskin. But the hood can be pulled back

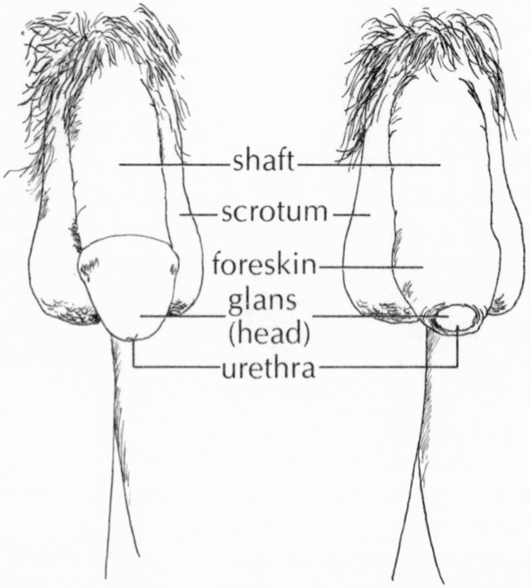

CIRCUMCISED PENIS (left) with glans entirely visible
UNCIRCUMCISED PENIS (right) with foreskin covering glans

to expose the head, and when erection occurs, the head naturally emerges. In fact, it's usually hard to tell whether or not a penis has been circumcised when it's erect. So it really doesn't make much difference in sexual activity.

The Testicles

The testicles are the two sperm-producing glands—the male counterpart of the female ovaries. They hang in a sack of crinkly skin called the scrotum. In most men it's normal for one testicle to hang a little lower—usually the left one.

The testicles are delicate organs. They are easily hurt if touched too hard, but they're capable of giving a lot of sexual pleasure if handled gently.

The testicles are highly susceptible to variations of heat and cold. The reason they hang in a sack outside the body, instead of being up inside in a more protected location, is that the heat of body temperature would kill the sperm they produce. Hanging outside the body keeps the testicles cooler.

Normally, when you're not sexually excited, the testicles move around inside the scrotum, and the shape of the scrotum changes continuously. If you're relaxed and warm, the balls hang loosely. If you're cold or nervous, the balls pull up closer to the body to conserve heat and protect themselves. You can see this yourself when you sit in a warm bathtub or swim in cold water.

Although the penis is the center of sexual excitement, the balls also react to stimulation. As soon as sexual excitement starts, the scrotum begins to tighten, and the testicles begin to rise. This action continues until the balls are hard and tight against the body.

As soon as you become sexually aroused, several glands swing into action and start producing liquid secretions. Usually when a man is highly excited, several drops of clear liquid are secreted from the tip of the penis. This corresponds to the female secretions in the vaginal walls during sexual arousal, and it's designed as a lubricant to ease the way into the vagina.

As sexual excitement grows, the penis becomes stiff and full, and the scrotum contracts in a tight round ball. When you're about to come, glands inside the body start releasing fluids and sperm that make up the semen.

At the moment of orgasm semen is forced through the urethra and out the penis by a series of rapid muscular contractions.

Afterwards everything begins to relax. The penis gets soft, the scrotum loosens, and the testicles begin to descend. It's all over until the next time.

Once a man has had an orgasm, it takes awhile before he can get sexually aroused again. Women can continue to have sex after they come, in fact, a woman can have two or three orgasms in a row. But a man's body always goes through a resting period after orgasm.

Sometimes this resting period lasts only a few minutes, sometimes it lasts a few hours. In either case, the body is simply giving itself a chance to unwind before sexual tension can build up again.

The Anus

The contractions in the penis during orgasm are always accompanied by spasmodic contractions at the same time in the anus. You can feel this yourself by putting a finger in your ass when you come.

The anus, by the way, is richly supplied with nerve endings like the penis, and it's capable of sexual stimulation. A lot of people are too uptight to think about the anus as part of their sexual anatomy, but using the ass can heighten sexual pleasure.

The prostate gland lies alongside the rectum, about four inches inside the body. It produces part of the liquid that makes up a man's semen. If you've ever been examined for some malfunction in the urinary system, you know a doctor can stick his finger in your rectum and make you come by massaging the back of the prostate gland. It doesn't feel very sexually exciting the way doctors do it—in fact, it hurts—but it will make you come. It's kind of like shortcutting the external machinery and going directly to the starter button.

The Chest

One area of the male body that's not usually thought of as sexually responsive is the chest. Actually a man's nipples contain clusters of nerve endings that make them sensitive and sexually excitable. Men's nipples, just like their female counterpart, get crinkled when they're cold, and they get erect during sexual excitement.

Not all men are sexually sensitive in their nipples, and many men never even notice their nipples because they think of breasts as exclusively feminine organs. But they're not. So if your nipples are sensitive, there's no reason not to enjoy them.

IT ALL WORKS TOGETHER

The way the body reacts to sex can seem very complicated. So many parts of you are doing different things at the same time. But when you're sexually excited, your body is acting spontaneously and naturally, and all of your sexual organs are working together.

For example, all the parts of a woman's genitals affect each other during sexual arousal. When something moves in and out of the vagina, it pulls the inner lips back and forth and stimulates the clitoris. If a woman gets turned on by just rubbing the clitoris, the vagina will still expand, secrete lubrication, and undergo contractions during orgasm.

Stroking a man's testicles will create pleasurable sensations that he also feels in his penis. In fact, no matter where the sexual stimulation is coming from, a man will feel it primarily in his penis, and a woman will feel it primarily in her clitoris.

The way your body responds to sex is always the same regardless of how you get excited. Fucking, fondling, or just thinking about sex will produce the same physical reactions in your gentials.

And the genitals aren't the only parts of you that react to sexual excitement. You breathe faster, your heart speeds up, and your blood flows faster. The muscles from head to feet become tense, and the whole body may perspire and become flushed.

Sex involves every part of you. And the more you get into your body, the more pleasure you'll find in it.

3

MASTURBATION

Masturbation is the act of stimulating your own body for sexual pleasure. It feels good, and it's perfectly natural.

Years ago people thought masturbation caused everything from pimples to insanity. Today we're told it will make us self-centered and neurotic.

All of that is bullshit. The only thing that will drive you crazy is not masturbating when your body wants to.

Masturbation won't make warts grow on your hands or cause your hair to fall out. In fact, doctors have found that masturbation is good for you. It provides a healthy release for sexual tension, and shrinks often recommend it for people who are sexually uptight. Sometimes women find that masturbating can even relieve their menstrual cramps.

And masturbation is one of the best ways to learn about your body and how it responds to sexual pleasure. You can read all the books in the world, but they can't tell you how your own body really feels. You've got to find that out for yourself.

There are lots of myths about masturbation. And most of them are designed to make us afraid of exploring our bodies.

Some people think that masturbation will change the way their genitals look. Women have been told that masturbating will make the clitoris grow longer or make the vaginal lips big and flabby. Some men think they can make their penis bigger by jerking off. All of this is nonsense. Masturbation, even lots and lots of it, has no physical effect on the size or shape of the genitals. That was all determined by nature, and there's not much we can do about it one way or the other.

Some people worry about masturbating too much. But there's really no such thing. Everybody's sexual appetite is different. If you masturbate three times a day, it's only a sign that you've got a strong sex drive. When your body has had enough, it will stop responding for a while, that's all.

Most people start masturbating long before they've had sex with anybody else, and nobody stops just because they've gotten laid. Masturbation is something people do all their lives.

And everybody does it—whether they like to admit it or not. Masturbation is a normal part of a normal sex life, even when you're having other kinds of sex.

Some people may think that masturbating isn't really part of sex, that it's just something to do when you can't find a partner. That's ridiculous. Sex starts with our own bodies. We masturbate because it feels good and because our bodies often need it.

Besides, masturbation is good preparation for having sex with another person. From touching yourself you can discover how and where you like to be stimulated, and that makes it easier to show someone else. It even makes it easier to learn how to touch and stimulate your partner's body.

Through masturbation you can also teach yourself how to reach orgasm quickly or how to delay your climax. That can be helpful in any kind of sexual relationship.

Society and our parents have made all of us feel a little guilty or embarrassed about masturbating. But it's important to remember that masturbation is the most common sexual practice in the world. We should all be able to talk about it—and enjoy it—like any other natural part of sex.

MASTURBATION AND MEN

Masturbation is something that comes naturally to most men. You start getting erections and strong sexual desires, and your body wants some kind of sexual release. Even if you ignore this appetite, you'll start having orgasms in your sleep. And any man who's had a wet dream will soon start trying to produce the sensations of orgasm when he's awake.

Men are also more accustomed to handling their own genitals than women, since a man has got to touch himself every time he takes a piss. And because the penis is such an obvious feature of the male body—and erections make it even more noticeable—it's perfectly natural for men to start touching themselves to get sexual pleasure.

But almost all men are reluctant to admit they masturbate. Somehow it's considered unmanly. Which is stupid, considering that men probably masturbate more than women.

In our society men are taught not to think about themselves as sexual creatures. Their attention is directed toward women's bodies. Men are supposed to be tough and careless about themselves; they're not supposed to go around stroking their bodies and giving themselves pleasure.

Men are also reluctant to talk about masturbation because it seems to reflect on their ability to have sex with women. A man masturbates, the argument goes, because he can't get laid.

The truth of the matter is that whether or not they have sex with other people, all men masturbate. And there's nothing unmasculine about it. Even cavemen, who seduced their women with clubs, probably jerked off.

Besides, sometimes there just isn't a partner around when you feel like having sex. And other times you may prefer to masturbate. That's not crazy, it's perfectly normal. Most people feel that way at times, and most people learn to enjoy their own company.

The urge to masturbate can come from anywhere—from looking at a *Playboy* centerfold, from erotic daydreams, or from just being horny.

How often you feel like masturbating depends on a lot of

things. You may get the urge to masturbate once a month, or you may feel like doing it three times a day. Both are normal, and everyone experiences different sex drives at different times.

The simplest way to masturbate is to pump the shaft of the erect penis up and down with your hand. By the speed and pressure of your stroking, you can control the sexual excitement. Although the term jerking off is used loosely to mean any kind of masturbation, it really describes this method best.

Another common method is to use some kind of lubrication. It makes masturbation feel more like intercourse, and it reduces the amount of work involved. Almost anything from soap to salad oil can be used, but commercial lubricants like vaseline are probably most popular—at least they won't irritate the penis.

Usually it takes only one hand to jerk off, and that leaves your other hand free. Holding your testicles, touching your thighs, or playing with any other part of your body will help increase sexual tension to the point of orgasm. If you find that your nipples are sensitive, or your ass, you can also use these parts of your body in masturbation.

Not all masturbating is done with the hands. Men have used every kind of object that they can fit their penis into. In fact, there's an entire industry that manufactures plastic vaginas for men to masturbate with.

No matter how you do it, the most noticeable part of jerking off is always the ejaculation—sperm and seminal fluid squirting out of the end of the penis. How much liquid is ejaculated depends on when you last came and how excited you are at the moment. To a certain extent the body stores up semen. If you haven't had any sexual release in a week, your ejaculation will probably be bigger than if you just came an hour ago.

Sometimes ejaculating can be a problem, especially if you want to keep your masturbating private. Maybe that's why many men jerk off in the bathroom where it's easy to dispose of the evidence. But the bathroom is a rather antiseptic and sexless place—nobody would think of doing all their fucking in the john.

If you're worried about coming all over the place and you don't want to get the sheets and towels stained, you might try masturbating in a rubber condom. It's easy to dispose of.

There must be hundreds of different ways to bring yourself to orgasm. So do whatever feels good, and don't worry about whether your method is "normal" or "masculine." Jerking off is the one sexual activity that all men have in common.

MASTURBATION AND WOMEN

Women used to pretend that masturbating was a male activity. "Nice girls" weren't supposed to need sex or even think about it very much. Women were supposed to think about getting married and using their bodies to have children.

But at some point every woman becomes aware of her own strong sex drive. And a healthy woman will begin to experiment with it.

Through masturbation you get to know your sexual moods —the times when your body is easily aroused and the times when it isn't. You learn how your body responds to different kinds of sexual sensations—what feels good and what doesn't. You become familiar with the physical changes your body goes through during sex. And you learn about your own orgasms.

Women often need practice with sex before they can have an orgasm during intercourse. And masturbation is the best kind of practice you can have.

Studies done on female sexuality show that women who masturbate can reach orgasm more easily and more frequently when they start balling than women who don't masturbate. And doctors specializing in sexual problems use masturbation as a treatment for women who have a hard time coming.

When you masturbate, you can really relax and get into your own body. You don't have to worry about how you look to your partner, whether you're pleasing him, or if your birth-control method will work. And you can take all the time you need to become stimulated.

Through experimenting and following your own instincts you can figure out what produces the most pleasure in your body. It's difficult for a man, even if he's very experienced, to know exactly what's going to feel best to you. Every woman is different. You've got to know yourself so you can show your partner.

In the privacy of your bedroom or when you're relaxing in the bathtub, you can start exploring your body by touching yourself all over.

You can learn how sensitive your breasts are by stroking and rubbing them. It may feel good when they're fondled very gently, or you may prefer more vigorous handling. You can play with the nipples and see if they crinkle up and become erect.

Some women don't find any particular erotic pleasure in stimulating their breasts, while others can have an orgasm that way without ever touching their genitals. And all women find that from time to time their breasts become so tender that only the most gentle caressing will feel good.

Since the clitoris is the center of a woman's sexual excitement, most women concentrate on that area when they masturbate, rather than the inside of the vagina.

Because it's so sensitive, it's sometimes more pleasurable to stimulate the clitoris indirectly. If you press against your pubic mound or rub the outer vaginal lips, you'll also feel the pleasurable sensations in your clitoris. As you become more aroused, you may want to massage yourself more vigorously or press directly against the clitoris, rubbing harder and faster until you come.

You may want to insert something into your vagina while you masturbate. Since the ring of muscle which forms the first third of the vagina is a very sensitive part of your sexual anatomy, the friction of something plunging in and out of your vagina as you massage your clitoris can add to your excitement.

The best thing to use is your own finger. It's convenient, it won't hurt your insides, and you can touch yourself in whatever way you want.

Women do masturbate with other things besides their fingers—everything from hotdogs to hairbrushes. If putting something inside your vagina turns you on, there's no reason not to, as long as you're not stupid about it. Don't use anything sharp or breakable, and don't use an empty bottle—it's dangerous.

There are also commercial products manufactured for masturbation. The most popular is the electric vibrator, a plastic penis-shaped instrument sold in many drugstores as a "body massager."

The vibrator stimulates the clitoral area and can also be inserted into the vagina, and many women find that it produces almost instant orgasms. But a vibrator makes a lot of noise, so if you're living at home with your family it might not be very practical.

When you massage your genitals, the delicate skin can get a little irritated after a while. But your body supplies a natural lubricant during sex by secreting fluids through the vaginal walls. If you put your finger inside your vagina, you can draw out some fluid to coat the clitoris.

No two women masturbate the exact same way. It's pretty much an instinct, and you learn quickly what feels best to you. The point is to get to know your own body as thoroughly as you can.

USING YOUR HEAD

Not all the pleasure of masturbation comes from your hands. Some of it comes from your head.

Daydreaming about sex can be a very pleasant activity. Thinking about someone else's body, or your own, or imagining sexual activity can get anyone turned on. Most students, in fact, spend at least a third of their time in class thinking about sex.

Sexual fantasies are a natural part of life, we even have them in our sleep. And almost everybody fantasizes when they masturbate.

Some people have very simple fantasies—like recalling a sexual pleasure from the past or thinking about one in the future. Other people construct complex scenes in which they're playing an imaginary role. In rare cases some people can fantasize so vividly that they reach orgasm without ever touching their genitals.

For most of us, however, fantasies just help to start and to heighten sexual arousal. It's perfectly normal to fantasize while you're masturbating, and everybody does it.

But most people also worry about their fantasies. They wonder if there's something wrong with them because of the sexual scenes they dream up. The whole point about fantasies, however, is that they're not real. They allow us to taste something we don't have or to experience a novel sexual situation without any of the real dangers or inhibitions involved.

It's perfectly natural to imagine that someone else is touching you when you're stimulating yourself. Men often imagine that their own hand is a vagina, and women sometimes fantasize that their finger is a penis.

Fantasies are frequently more exciting when they center around some activity that we'd be afraid to do in real life.

For example, homosexual fantasies are very common for both men and women. They don't mean that you're a homosexual or even that you'd enjoy a real homosexual experience.

People fantasize about being raped, or about masturbating in front of an audience or about having sex with a close relative.

None of these is sick—in fact, they're pretty routine. They show only that thinking about something forbidden can be sexually exciting. And the more experience people have had, the more unusual their fantasies are liable to become.

But whatever your sexual fantasies, don't worry about them. An active imagination can make masturbation more fun. In fact, it can make all of your sex life more fun. And you've got every right to explore your own head, just as you have every right to explore your own body.

4

LOSING YOUR VIRGINITY

A virgin is someone who's never had intercourse—and that can be either a man or a woman. You can have a lot of sexual experience from masturbating, making out, even oral sex, and still technically be a virgin.

In our society most people are forced to wait several years or longer after they've become physically ready to have intercourse. And during that time all kinds of anxieties get built up about balling. What should be one of the most natural and enjoyable events of our lives becomes a monumental hurdle we have to jump over.

For a woman, losing her virginity can be a complicated experience. There can be emotional issues as well as physical problems involved in it.

For a man, having intercourse for the first time isn't really a physical hassle, but there can be other problems caused by lack of familiarity with a woman's body.

Some people may lose their virginity in a moment of unplanned passion, other people are very deliberate and careful. But no matter how casual or carried away people seem, almost everybody is nervous about fucking for the first time.

And it's important for both men and women to tell your partner if you're a virgin. A lot of people feel insecure about being sexually inexperienced and like to sound as if they've been around a bit more than they really have. But everybody starts out being a virgin, and everybody has to go through the experience of balling for the first time.

Telling your partner can relieve a lot of suspense and anxiety. Maybe your partner is a virgin too, and talking about it will make both of you feel a lot more secure with each other. If you're losing your virginity with someone who's already had intercourse, your partner can help you.

A lot of people go through awkward experiences that are totally unnecessary just because they refused to mention their virginity. But if you're going to have sex with someone, it only makes sense to start off being honest.

Whether you're having intercourse for the first time yourself or you're having sex with someone who is a virgin, there are a few practical things like the hymen and birth control that have to be considered in advance.

THE HYMEN

A woman's hymen is usually made out to be a much bigger deal than it really is. Most people think you can always tell whether or not a woman is a virgin by her hymen. But that's not really true.

The hymen is a thin web of tissue about one-half inch inside the vaginal opening, partially closing off the vagina. There are holes in the hymen, which make it easier to puncture than a solid piece of skin.

Not all women have a hymen to begin with. And by the time many women get around to fucking, the hymen is already stretched from using tampons or broken by a finger during masturbation or making out. Even leading a physically active life can break the fragile hymen.

If a woman's hymen is still intact when she gets laid for the first time, the penis tears a hole in it when it enters the vagina. Repeated intercourse continues to erode the hymen until nothing is left but a little ring of tissue that often remains around the vaginal opening throughout a woman's whole life.

Breaking the skin of the hymen sometimes hurts a little, and the small blood vessels in the hymen may bleed for a while. But most stories about losing virginity greatly exaggerate the pain and bleeding, probably to discourage women from getting laid.

Some women don't feel anything when their hymen is broken. Other women feel a sharp kind of pain that is over in a couple of seconds. As for the bleeding, you probably won't even notice it until intercourse is over.

If a woman is curious about the state of her hymen, she can examine herself by putting a finger in her vaginal opening and feeling for a piece of tissue blocking the inside of the vagina.

If you can run your finger from the vaginal lips to deep inside the vagina with no obstruction, either the hymen is not intact or it's stretched wide enough that your finger can get through a hole in it. That means a penis can get through too with a little extra push.

Since the hymen is so small, and since a woman may not be familiar enough with her body to find it, you can't always be sure by examining yourself. But this might give you some idea about what to expect in having intercourse for the first time.

BIRTH CONTROL

A lot of men and women say that losing their virginity was an accident, something that "just happened." They didn't know they were going to fuck when they started making out. In fact, so many people are intent upon their first experience being a spontaneous act of love and passion that they don't want to make any kind of preparation for it at all.

This is very romantic—but very stupid. Women can and do get pregnant the first time they have intercourse, especially women who insist on being spontaneous and natural.

In fact, a woman can get pregnant any time she has intercourse. She's not automatically safe just because she's having her period. And she's definitely not safe just because the man withdraws his penis before he comes.

The drops of lubricating fluid that form on the tip of a man's penis when he's sexually excited usually contain small amounts of sperm. And just by inserting the penis a little way inside the vagina, it's possible for a woman to get pregnant even though the man hasn't ejaculated.

So birth control is something you need any time and every time you have intercourse.

There are many kinds of birth control that you can get easily and cheaply. For more detailed information about each kind of birth control, how they work, and how to get them, see Chapter 10.

A woman doesn't have to be married to get some kind of birth control, and she can go to a doctor or birth-control clinic even if she's a virgin. But don't borrow something like a diaphragm or birth-control pills from a friend. Chances are they won't be right for your body.

Condoms and spermicidal foams are available to both men and women in most drugstores. And if you don't take the trouble to get anything else, you should at least have condoms.

Sometimes people hesitate to go out and get birth control because they find it embarrassing. A man may feel uncomfortable going into a crowded drugstore and asking for rubbers. A woman may not want to go to a doctor or clinic because she's afraid they'll disapprove of her intention to have sex. So what if they give you a funny look? It's your body.

Having intercourse for the first time can make you nervous enough without having to worry about an accidental pregnancy all the way through it.

FIRST INTERCOURSE

There are lots of things a man and woman can do to make first intercourse easier. Being sensitive to your partner's body and helping each other will make losing your virginity more fun.

Making out prepares your body naturally for intercourse. The more you kiss, stroke, and caress each other's bodies and genitals, the more sexually excited you become. Women usually take a little longer to get sexually aroused, so a man shouldn't think that as soon as he's got an erection, his partner is ready too. The fact is that a man can get an erection in five seconds, but it may take a woman five minutes—or much longer—to be equally excited.

When you're making out, it's a good idea for a man to put his finger inside the woman's vagina. If a woman is nervous, she may unconsciously contract her vaginal muscle as her whole body tenses up, which will make it harder for the man's penis to enter her. By working his finger around, the man can stretch and relax the vaginal opening. The woman will be more sexually ready for a penis if she's entered by something smaller first.

Inserting a finger will also help the man get used to the position and angle of his partner's vagina. It's liable to stretch or tear an intact hymen, but intercourse is much easier for both the man and the women if the hymen is stretched by a finger before it's stretched by a penis.

The man can also draw out some of the woman's internal secretions with his finger to lubricate her vaginal opening. Men and women produce natural lubricants when they're excited, but a woman may not lubricate much if she's nervous.

Sometimes it's a good idea, although it requires a lot of foresight, to use something like vaseline. It may cut down on the spontaneity to stop and apply lubrication, but it will also make it much easier for the penis to get into the vagina.

Many kinds of condoms are already lubricated. If you're going to use condoms for birth control, it's a good idea to choose lubricated ones if the woman is a virgin.

People can fuck in a lot of different ways, but the position most people choose for their first intercourse is the traditional one, with the woman lying on her back and the man on top.

In this position the woman should spread her legs and pull her knees up. This will raise her vagina and make it easier

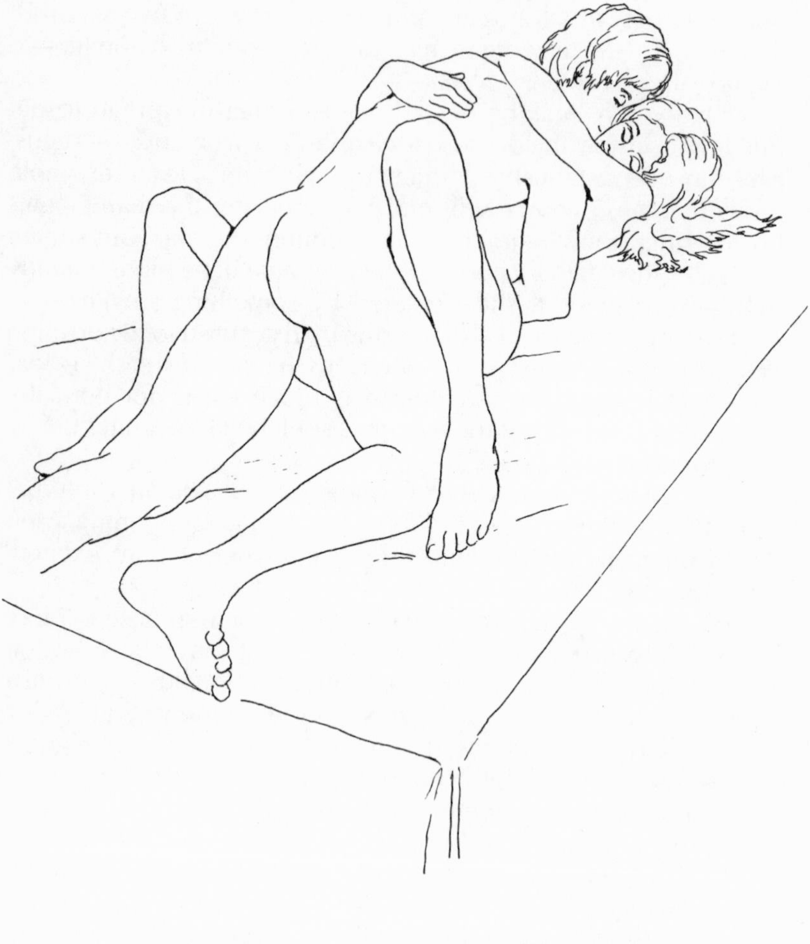

for the penis to enter. Men sometimes push at the wrong angle when they're having intercourse for the first time. But the woman can help by guiding the man's penis into her vagina with her hands.

If the woman's hymen is intact, the man may find that he can enter the vagina only a little bit before running up against resistance. When he feels the resistance of the hymen, he's going to have to push through it, firmly but gently. It's not a good idea to thrust the penis into the vagina in one swift plunge. That can cause a woman pain.

It's better to push the penis in against the hymen and then pull back a little, pushing more forcefully each time. That helps open the entrance to the vagina, and the lubricating fluids will be spread around. And at the same time, the woman should be making an effort to relax her vaginal muscle rather than squeezing it tight, and lifting her pelvis toward her partner as he pushes into her.

Once the penis has gotten all the way into the vagina, it's best to stop for a minute, so the woman can get used to the feeling of having a penis inside her. Then the man can start moving his penis slowly back and forth while the woman pushes her pelvis toward him, moving an inch or two at first and gradually making the movements longer and faster.

At this point you've made it.

Chances are a man losing his virginity will reach orgasm a lot faster than he expects. And chances are a woman having intercourse for the first time won't reach orgasm at all. Most women need a little experience with the sensations of intercourse before they can have orgasms while they're fucking.

But there's no reason why a man shouldn't make a woman come with his hand by massaging and stroking her clitoris. After all, the idea of sex is mutual pleasure, and it's not a woman's fault if it takes her longer and she has to go through more discomfort losing her virginity than a man does.

A lot of women don't realize that the semen the man ejaculated inside her—if he hasn't worn a condom—is going to come out. It may spill out of your vagina as soon as the man withdraws his penis, or it may not come out until after you've been walking around for a while. So if you suddenly feel something sticky trickling down your leg, don't panic.

A woman's vagina may hurt for a while if she just lost her virginity, in fact, it may be sore for a few days. That's perfectly normal. But if both of you feel like fucking again, there's no reason not to. It's always better the second time.

THE MORNING AFTER

It may be a hassle, it may even be disappointing, but most people are glad about losing their virginity.

In fact, it's usually a relief to have it over with. Now you're free to choose whatever kind of sexual activity and whatever kind of relationship you want.

Like anything else, fucking gets better with practice. Women usually learn how to respond more rapidly, and men usually learn how to slow down. Repeated intercourse, especially with the same partner, brings greater mutual pleasure.

People sometimes wonder if their lack of virginity is obvious to anyone else. There are lots of old stories to the effect that people look different after they begin fucking, that women who aren't virgins walk differently, or that your parents will take one look at you and know immediately. That's all nonsense. No physical change takes place when you have intercourse that anybody else could ever see.

The only thing different about you may be a new sense of self-confidence about your own body and your own sexuality. And that feels good.

5

FEMALE ORGASM

Orgasm is a very similar feeling for both women and men. When sexual excitement has built up to a very high level, the genitals contract in a series of spasms, and a wave of sexual pleasure and release flows through the whole body.

But there are some important differences between the male and female body. When a man comes, it's very noticeable—semen is ejaculated from the end of his penis. When a woman reaches orgasm, her physical reaction is less visible and not as easy to pinpoint. And this difference has contributed to a lot of confusion and misunderstanding about the female orgasm.

When people start having intercourse regularly, a man finds that reaching orgasm for him is a fairly simple matter. His body gets aroused easily, and he can come quickly.

A woman, on the other hand, may find that she's not reaching orgasm at all during intercourse. Even women who have had several orgasms from masturbating or making out may not come when they begin to fuck.

Most people don't understand the difference between male and female sexual response. They expect a woman to react to sex just like a man. And when she doesn't, both the man and woman usually start wondering what's wrong.

A man may think he's a lousy lover if the woman he's making it with doesn't have an orgasm. And a woman may worry about whether there's something wrong with her physically or psychologically.

And it's hard for a young woman to get the kind of information she needs about her own sexuality. Parents are no help, and books are usually worse.

Sometimes a woman may have read so many exaggerated descriptions of what orgasm is supposed to be, with bells ringing, lights flashing, and the earth trembling, that when she does have an orgasm, she figures it can't be the real thing—it wasn't dramatic enough.

ONLY ONE KIND OF ORGASM

There are lots of misleading and distorted descriptions of the female orgasm floating around in books and magazines. Forty years ago Sigmund Freud thought up the idea that women could have two different kinds of orgasms—one in the clitoris and another in the vagina. In the last few years the women's liberation movement has produced a lot of writers who claim that vaginal orgasms don't exist, only clitoral orgasms.

Both the Freudians and the feminists are wrong. There is no such thing as separate vaginal or clitoral orgasms. There is only one kind of female orgasm, and it always involves both the clitoris and the vagina at the same time.

All modern sex studies, from the famous Kinsey report to the medical research of Masters and Johnson, have proven this. And any woman can feel it herself in her own body.

A woman's body will always go through the same physical changes and experience the same sensations of pleasure during orgasm regardless of whether the clitoris or the vagina or both are being stimulated. And although orgasms can vary in intensity, they're always basically the same for a woman, just as they're always basically the same for a man.

When a woman is sexually stimulated in any way—by having any part of her body kissed or touched—sexual excitement is communicated to the whole genital area, but the woman feels it most in her clitoris. The clitoris reacts to excitement by swelling. The vagina reacts by secreting lubrication, and the vaginal lips swell and spread apart.

During orgasm the muscular outer third of the vagina begins contracting in quick spasms, and a throbbing sensation of pleasure spreads through the entire genital area.

It doesn't matter whether the orgasm is a result of masturbating or balling or oral sex, or whether it happens during heterosexual or homosexual activity. Feelings of arousal will always build up in the clitoris, and the vagina will always undergo contractions.

If you massage the clitoris without having anything inside the vagina, vaginal contractions will still take place during orgasm. And if you're balling, the clitoris always gets excited even if you don't touch it, because sexual feeling from the rest of your genitals is communicated to the clitoris.

But an orgasm is an experience that involves the whole body—not just the clitoris and the vagina. The uterus and sometimes the anus undergo contractions along with the vagina, and muscles throughout your body jump around. As orgasm ends, pleasurable sensations of release are spread through the whole body.

If a woman has had one orgasm, she's had the only kind there is. And if a woman can come when she's masturbating, she can come during intercourse. It's just a question of learning how.

HAVING AN ORGASM

If a woman wants to have an orgasm, the easiest thing to do is masturbate.

Find a nice comfortable place and try stimulating your own body. Concentrate on exciting your clitoris. When you come, the sensations of pleasure will spread out from your clitoris through your whole genital area. If you put a finger inside your vagina you can feel the orgasmic contractions.

Masturbation is a good way to reach orgasm, because you can really relax and give yourself all the stimulation you need. By experimenting you'll discover what feels best to your body.

If you want to have an orgasm during intercourse, you've got to get enough stimulation on your sensitive clitoris.

First of all, you should make sure your partner excites your body before intercourse. If you start to fuck before your body is ready, your partner may come before you're even aroused.

Any position for intercourse will provide some clitoral stimulation. During intercourse the penis tugs at the inner lips of the vagina, and this pulls on the clitoris. But for many women that's just not enough. So choose a position that brings your clitoris into direct contact with the man's pubic area. Or one that allows your partner to stimulate your genitals with his hand while you're fucking.

It's also important for a woman to use her body actively during intercourse. Rub your genitals against your partner's body, or take his hand and show him where you want to be touched.

Or you can use your own hands during intercourse. If you're fucking in the traditional position with the man on top, it's easier for you to touch your clitoris than for your partner. You might think it's embarrassing, but there's no reason it should be. After all, the point of sex is not just to give your partner pleasure but to give yourself pleasure too.

One of the major differences between male and female sexual response is that a woman can have a second orgasm soon after she's had her first. A man can't. After he comes, his body goes through a waiting period before he can get sexually aroused again. A woman doesn't have to wait at all. She can be brought to orgasm again with more stimulation.

Some women can have several orgasms, one right after another. This series of little orgasms, separated by only a few seconds, is called multiple orgasm. Most women, though, have only one orgasm during sex. That's all they need to feel perfectly satisfied.

If you really want to have an orgasm during intercourse, it

helps to talk with your partner. Most people are embarrassed to talk about their sexual responses, and women especially rely on their partner to figure out what gives them pleasure.

But men aren't born with any automatic knowledge about how a woman's body feels. And if a woman is too shy to talk about her sexual preferences, there's no way her partner is ever going to find out.

There are lots of ways a woman can reach orgasm, and when you feel comfortable talking about sex, you can feel more comfortable experimenting.

HAVING TROUBLE

Besides knowing how women have orgasms, it's important to understand why they don't.

The most common reason a woman doesn't reach orgasm during intercourse is that she hasn't gotten enough sexual stimulation. Some women need a lot of direct clitoral contact, other women need to have intercourse for a long time. In either case, the problem can be solved if the woman explains her sexual needs to her partner and uses her body actively during intercourse to get the kind of stimulation she wants.

Often there can be a very simple reason why a woman doesn't reach orgasm. If she's fucking without any kind of birth control, she will probably be preoccupied with fears of pregnancy. And that interferes with physical pleasure. If a woman is making it in the back seat of a car, sex may be too hurried for her to get excited. If she's at home expecting her parents to walk in any second, a woman may be too nervous about being discovered to get into the sexual experience.

Sometimes there are more complicated reasons that prevent a woman from reaching orgasm.

All of us grow up with some kind of guilt about sex that filters down from our parents or from society. If a woman feels guilty, she may inhibit herself from having orgasms—even without realizing it.

Some women feel that they have to be in love with their partner in order to enjoy sex. If a woman is too hung up on worrying about love instead of concentrating on her sexual pleasure while she's fucking, she may not be able to come.

Sometimes a woman can be so concerned with whether or not she'll have an orgasm that she makes it impossible to have one. A woman who doesn't come as soon as she starts balling might not realize how common that situation is. She's liable to think there's something wrong with her and worry about that instead of getting into sex and digging the pleasure.

Women who can't have orgasms are often called frigid. Technically, being frigid means that a woman is totally incapable of getting any physical pleasure out of sex. But the word is seldom used correctly. More often than not, it's just a sexual insult, like calling somebody a prude or a faggot.

Real frigidity is very rare. There are some women who never experience orgasm throughout a whole life of active sexual relations. But even these women are not necessarily frigid. Usually there's some block that stands in the way of their sexual fulfillment—and it's just a matter of getting around it.

Basically a woman can have trouble reaching orgasm if anything is distracting her from enjoying her own body. If she's thinking about something else or if there's some problem lurking in the back of her mind, her physical response can be inhibited. To really enjoy sex, you've got to relax and get into yourself.

But a woman who's just discovering her own sexuality should remember that lack of experience is probably her biggest problem. You can't expect to be thoroughly familiar with the new sensations of intercourse overnight. And it takes time for two people to learn each other's bodies.

With a healthy attitude, a little practice, and a considerate partner, you can get all the pleasure you want out of sex.

FAKING IT

Women sometimes fake orgasm when they're having intercourse. By pretending that she's getting more and more excited, breathing heavily, groaning, and jerking her pelvis back and forth, a woman can almost always get away with making a man think she's come.

The question is, why would any woman want to?

Sometimes a woman fakes orgasm to please her partner. A man may take a woman's orgasm as proof of his own sexual skill, and a woman fakes orgasm to reassure her partner and not disappoint him.

Women also fake orgasm because they feel embarrassed at not having one. Most women take the orgasm as proof of their own sexuality, and not reaching orgasm might be the same as admitting a lack of womanliness.

But faking orgasms is a lousy thing to do. In terms of your relationship with another person, it's just lying with your body. A woman who fakes orgasm may think she's fooling her partner, but she's only cheating herself. It makes more sense to concentrate on the real pleasure your body is feeling than to get hung up on pretending.

It's important for both men and women to realize that not all women reach orgasm every time they fuck. That's perfectly normal. A woman's body feels and reacts differently at different times.

Sometimes having sex without orgasm can be frustrating for a woman. But other times it can be perfectly satisfying. There's a lot of physical pleasure and emotional closeness in sex, and for many women this is just as important as having an orgasm.

Orgasm isn't an isolated event. It's a result of sexual pleasure. If a woman is relaxed about sex, if she enjoys the sexual feelings in her own body, then orgasm will come about naturally.

6

INTERCOURSE

Fucking is a natural instinct. Any kind of sexual stimulation, whether it's kissing, caressing, or just thinking about sex, automatically starts preparing your body to have intercourse. A man's penis gets erect, and a woman's vagina begins to get wet.

But there's more to sexual intercourse than just putting a penis inside a vagina. That's only the beginning. Every time you have sex you learn more about how to use your body and how to share sexual pleasure.

The pleasure of intercourse depends on how you use your entire body, not on the size or shape of your sex organs. Many people think that fucking is better if the man has a large cock and the woman has a small vagina. But that's a myth. The fact is that everybody's sexual organs are perfectly well suited for each other.

The average penis is five or six inches long when erect. But the average vagina is only about four inches long—it's got to expand during intercourse to accommodate the penis.

It's true that one woman's vagina may feel larger than another's, but that's usually the result of vaginal lubrication. If a woman secretes a lot of lubricating fluid when she's excited, her vagina will be easier to enter and may even feel "roomier" than a woman whose vagina is drier. But that feeling has nothing to do with size, since any woman's vagina can expand or contract to fit almost any size penis.

Besides, the most sensitive part of a woman's vagina is the outer third. And the most sensitive part of the penis is the head. So with just the head of the penis moving an inch or two inside the vagina, both the man and the woman are going to get plenty of sexual stimulation.

Pushing the penis deeper into the vagina, however, produces different sensations. As a man moves in and out he can feel the vagina stroke the entire length of his penis. And for a woman deep penetration brings the man's pubic area into contact with her sensitive vaginal lips and clitoris.

Many people also think that fucking is something a man does to a woman. It's not—fucking is something two people do with each other for mutual pleasure. A woman is just as free as a man to initiate sex, and her pleasure shouldn't depend exclusively on the man's performance. It also depends on how actively she seeks her own pleasure.

The vagina is not a passive receptacle. Any woman can use her vagina just as actively during intercourse as a man uses his penis. By thrusting her hips and swinging her pelvis, a woman not only excites her partner but also helps create the kind of stimulation she needs in the vagina and the clitoris to bring her to orgasm.

Some people think that a woman shouldn't fuck when she is having her period. That's nonsense. There will probably be a little menstrual blood inside the vagina, and the man might notice some on his penis afterward. But it's perfectly harmless, and it doesn't interfere with pleasure at all.

It's possible that a woman may find intercourse uncomfortable if she's having menstrual cramps. But often a woman is most sexually responsive just before and during her period. She may want to have sex more at that time, and it may feel better.

There's no physical reason why a man and woman can't fuck anytime they feel like it.

POSITIONS AND PLACES

There are lots of ways to have intercourse. You can do it with the man on top or the woman on top. You can fuck standing on your feet or standing on your head. It doesn't really matter—the pleasure is always going to be centered in your genitals. But different positions do allow you to touch and stimulate each other in different ways.

The most common way to fuck is face to face with the man lying on top of the woman. It's not always the best position for the woman to reach orgasm, but making out leads naturally to balling this way since it's easy to get the penis into the vagina.

Lying face to face, you can use your hands and mouths to kiss and caress each other. The man can play with the woman's breasts while she strokes his back or buttocks. All this adds to sexual pleasure.

There are lots of ways to move your body in this basic position. If the woman draws her knees up to her chest or rests her legs over the man's shoulders, the vagina is very accessible. The man can move in and out in long thrusts and the penis penetrates deeply into the vagina.

If the woman closes her legs inside the man's and squeezes her thighs together, the vagina will feel tighter around the penis. The woman gets added pleasure on her clitoris, and the man gets the extra stimulation of feeling his testicles pressed between the woman's thighs.

You can reverse the traditional male and female roles by having the man lie flat on his back while the woman lies on top of him. The woman has to take the lead, raising and lowering her vagina on the penis while the man moves his pelvis to meet her.

When the woman is lying on top, she has more control over the speed and rhythm of intercourse, and many women find this is the best position for clitoral stimulation. Besides that,

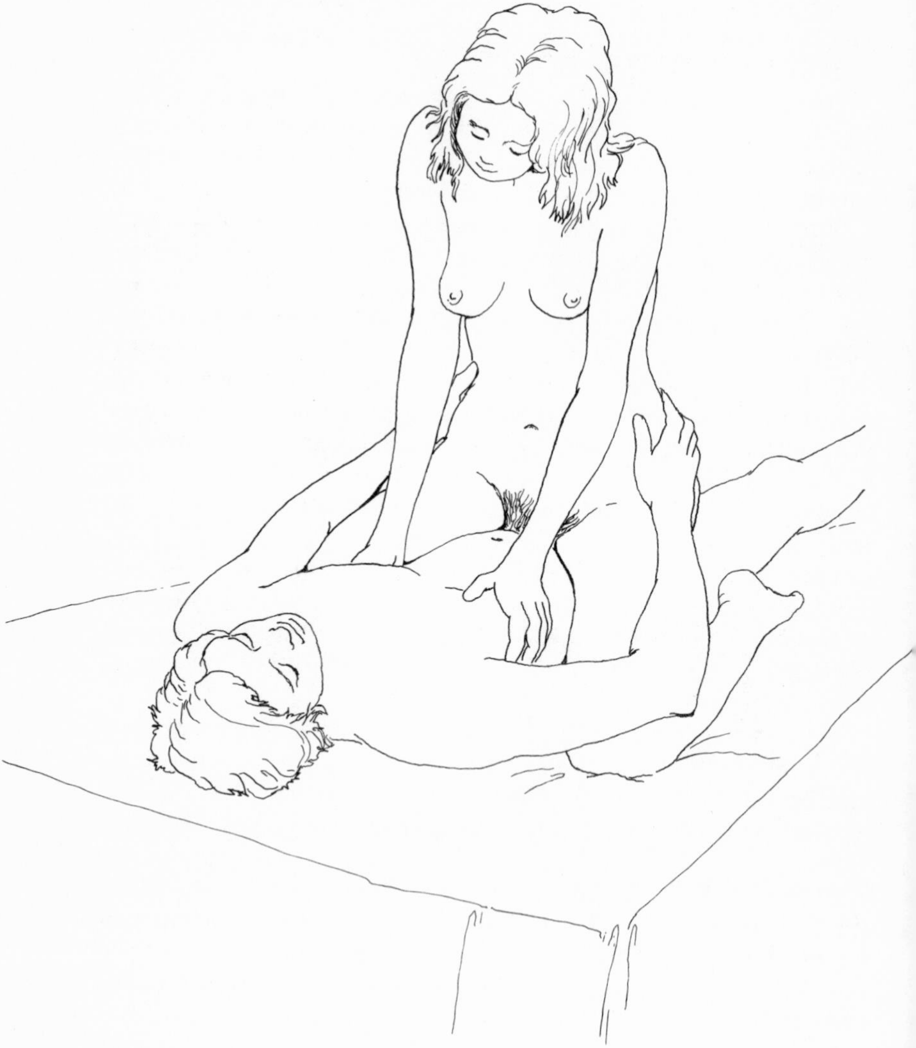

it's exciting for both the man and the woman to switch roles.

The only problem is that the penis can slip out of the vagina easily. But if the woman raises herself up to a sitting position on top of the man, the penis penetrates deeper into the vagina. And in this position you can see and touch most of each other's bodies.

You don't have to keep your eyes closed all the time you're having intercourse. In fact, it's sexy to open your eyes and look at each other. With the woman sitting on top of the man, you can both watch each other's expressions of pleasure.

Human beings are unique because they can have intercourse in so many positions. Most animals, for example, have only one way to fuck, and that's with the male mounting the female from behind. Men and women are also constructed to have intercourse this way, and it's perfectly natural.

If the woman leans forward on her hands and knees, the man can enter easily from behind, and the penis penetrates deep into the vagina. Although you can't see or kiss each other in this position, it offers other kinds of sexual sensations. The woman's buttocks rub against the man's whole pubic area, and with his hands free the man can stroke the woman's breasts or clitoris.

It's also fun to fuck sitting up, with the woman resting her weight on top of the man's thighs and her legs wrapped around his waist. In this position you're face to face, and you can both move your bodies together.

Or you can make it lying side by side. This position gives the woman good clitoral stimulation, but it's difficult for the man to get his penis into the vagina in this position. It's easier to start with one of you on top and then roll over on your sides.

In fact, you can always start in one position and then move on to another. Intercourse doesn't have to be a two-minute experience. The more time you take, the more intense your pleasure will be. Sometimes it feels best to just lie still and not move at all—just kiss and caress each other. It's possible to have intercourse for hours by just moving your genitals every once in a while to keep excited.

And intercourse doesn't have to be confined to bed either.

You can always make it in a chair, on the floor, or standing against a wall.

Finding a private place to fuck is often the most difficult problem of sex. But you can have intercourse practically anywhere—in a car, in a field, or up to your neck in water.

Balling in a car is pretty uncomfortable, but lots of people do it. However, it's best if the car is standing still and not zipping along at 90 mph.

Fucking outside in the woods or a field can be really beautiful. The sun, the wind, and the sky make you realize how much your body—and sex—are a part of the natural cycle of life.

And fucking in a lake or ocean is fun because your body is almost weightless. If the woman throws her legs around the man's hips, he can hold her weight easily and both of you can move freely.

One way of making it that's almost like intercourse doesn't involve putting the penis inside the vagina at all. The woman lies on her back and draws her knees up to her chest, and the man presses the underside of his penis flat against the vaginal lips—not inside the vagina but on top of it. As the man strokes back and forth, his penis caresses the woman's entire vulva.

Using some kind of artificial lubricant will reduce friction between the penis and the vaginal lips and will increase the sexual pleasure for both of you. A woman can reach orgasm quickly this way because the clitoris is being stimulated directly by the penis.

And when the man reaches orgasm, his ejaculation will spurt out on the woman's belly. Most women find it sexually exciting to see a man come—it's something they can't see when the penis is inside the vagina.

This is also a good way to make it if you're caught without any kind of birth control. Both of you can reach orgasm and you don't risk pregnancy—provided, of course, that the man ejaculates far enough away from the opening of the vagina.

The number of ways you can have intercourse depends only on your imagination and your energy. Couples who have sex with each other a lot usually find their own favorite variations.

COMING TOGETHER

One of the most popular myths about intercourse is thinking that if a man and woman have really good sex together, they'll reach orgasm at the same moment. Simultaneous orgasm is nice when it happens, but it doesn't happen all the time, even with experienced couples.

During intercourse a man gets the maximum sexual stimulation on his penis as it moves in and out of the vagina. So he can usually reach orgasm quickly.

But a woman gets only indirect stimulation on her clitoris during intercourse, and it will usually take her longer to reach orgasm. This is no reflection on the sexual ability of either partner. It's a simple fact of life.

Men and women are not built the same. But there are lots of things a man and woman can do together to make their sexual excitement more equal.

Spending a longer time making out can get a woman more sexually excited before the penis even enters the vagina.

During intercourse a man can stroke the clitoris with his hand or press against it with his pubic area.

Women can learn how to move their bodies to get the maximum stimulation where they need it.

And men can learn to hold back their orgasm so intercourse can last longer.

Just as some women have difficulty reaching orgasm, some men have difficulty restraining it. If a man comes as soon as his penis enters the vagina, it's probably because he's overeager. Sexual excitement has been built up to the point that the man is already on the verge of orgasm. And the feel of the vagina is the final erotic sensation needed to push him over the top.

Most young men tend to reach orgasm quickly, especially if they don't have sex with the same woman regularly. If you want to prolong intercourse, it's a good idea not to stimulate the penis too much before fucking.

After a man reaches orgasm, he usually can't go on fucking for very long. His body cools off as quickly as it warmed up.

The penis begins to go soft, and he has to wait for a while until he can be sexually aroused again. But if a man reaches orgasm first, he can always continue stimulating the woman with his hand or body.

A woman's sexual excitement builds more slowly than a man's, and she usually cools off at a much slower rate. If a woman reaches orgasm first, she can always keep on fucking until her partner comes too.

Male and female sexual responses are not identical. But once you get used to having intercourse, you learn what to expect from your own body and what to expect from your partner. It doesn't matter whether orgasm comes fast or slow, separately or simultaneously—it always feels good.

7

EXPANDING SEX

Having sex involves your entire body. Although sexual excitement is centered in the genitals, it's important to remember that the rest of the body is sexually sensitive too.

The belly, the buttocks, the thighs, are all highly erogenous areas in both men and women.

Stroking the back, the shoulders, or the legs can be very erotic. And it feels good to have your ears kissed or your neck or your nipples.

In fact, there's no part of the body that can't provide sexual pleasure. And using your hands and mouth during sex is just as important as using your genitals.

Your hands are really one of the most important parts of your sexual equipment. With your hands you can express affection, arouse sexual feelings, or bring your partner to orgasm.

All sexual activity from making out to fucking involves touching and stroking. And learning how to use your hands to give each other pleasure is something that takes understanding and practice.

Men can sometimes be too rough with their hands. Women can sometimes be too shy. If you're lying in bed naked, try caressing each other from head to foot. Explore every curve and fold with your fingers. Everybody likes back rubs, and body rubs are even better.

A woman needs to have her body stimulated to prepare her for intercourse. But there's more to making out than just grabbing the breasts or clitoris. Most women prefer being touched all over—gently and slowly.

A woman's breasts are made of delicate tissue, especially the nipples. Pinching or biting them too hard can produce more pain than pleasure. It's best for a man to cup the breast with his hand and rub the nipple lightly. As a woman becomes more sexually excited, her breasts can be squeezed more firmly.

The same is true for the clitoris. It's best to begin by stroking the whole pubic area, the thighs, and the vaginal lips. The clitoris itself needs to be handled gently—massaging the whole clitoris is more stimulating than pressing a finger into the sensitive glans.

Inserting a finger into the vagina feels good too. A man can use his finger like a penis while rubbing the vaginal lips and clitoris with the rest of his hand.

A man doesn't require as much preparation for intercourse as a woman does. All he needs is an erection, and a woman can always arouse a man by stroking his penis. But caressing his chest, his thighs, and the whole area around his genitals will produce even greater sexual excitement.

Although the penis is the most sexually sensitive part of a man's body, it's a pretty strong organ. You can squeeze it, shake it, bend it, or pull on it. That's not always the best way for a woman to handle a man's penis, but you don't have to be afraid of injuring it.

A woman can stroke the penis lightly with her fingertips or put her hand snugly around the shaft of the penis and pump up and down. Both feel good, but it's probably best to begin with slow gentle touches and gradually increase the pressure and speed of your stroking.

The balls are a different story. They have to be handled carefully. It's not the scrotum—the skin—that is so delicate, but the two testicles inside. Cupping the testicles in your hand and gently massaging them can be very exciting, especially if you're stroking the penis at the same time.

Touching each other doesn't have to be something you do only before or during intercourse—you can make it with your hands instead of fucking.

Bringing each other to orgasm with your hands is usually called mutual masturbation. But that's a wrong term, since it's not really masturbation at all. It's a form of sex that involves being sensitive to each other and knowing how to touch your partner's body to produce maximum pleasure.

ORAL SEX

The mouth is a very sexy part of your body. You use it to create and communicate sexual pleasure in a lot of ways—smiling, talking, kissing.

Kissing is such a natural thing that nobody makes a big deal about it. But the mouth is a sensitive erogenous zone. And when you bring two mouths together, you're both giving and getting erotic stimulation. Kissing can be almost like fucking with your mouth when you move your tongue back and forth to imitate the action of intercourse.

And if kissing someone's mouth feels good, kissing the rest of the body feels even better. It's very sensuous to kiss the neck or the nipples. And it's extremely exciting to put your mouth on each other's genitals.

When a woman uses her mouth on a man's genitals, it's called fellatio, and when a man does it to a woman, it's called cunnilingus. Both are just technical terms for giving head, sucking, eating, or going down on each other.

Kissing and sucking each other's genitals is a natural part of sex. Most people do it if they're not uptight about their bodies. Some people may hesitate to have oral sex because they think the genitals are dirty. But they're cleaner and more germ-free than your mouth.

Exciting each other's genitals with your mouth is something

you can do before intercourse, or you can bring each other to orgasm with your mouths instead of fucking. In either case, it's a very intimate way to have sex.

When a woman goes down on a man, she uses her mouth sort of like her vagina. Sucking the penis in and out of her mouth gives the man the same kind of stimulation as intercourse, massaging the penis from the tip all the way down the shaft.

There are lots of other ways a woman can use her mouth to give a man pleasure. She can take the penis out of her mouth and lick it with her tongue or suck on the head of the cock or rub her lips back and forth along the sensitive underside of the penis.

It also feels good if she uses her mouth and hands on the testicles. Kissing or stroking anywhere in the genital area is exciting. And pumping the penis with your hand while you suck on it will bring a man to orgasm very quickly.

The only problem a woman may have when she sucks the penis is keeping her teeth out of the way. A gentle nibble might feel good, but scraping the teeth along the cock is only going to hurt. And it may take a little practice to learn how to use your mouth without using your teeth.

When a man is about to come, his body may freeze for a second. But even though he stops moving, the woman shouldn't. The man will ejaculate his semen in a few spurts, and he'll get more pleasure if the woman keeps sucking throughout his whole orgasm.

And after he comes, it feels good if the woman holds the man's cock in her mouth while his body begins to relax.

The first few times a woman gives head, she may feel a little squeamish about swallowing the man's come. But semen is a natural substance, and it can't hurt you. In fact, it's actually good for you, since it's made up mostly of protein.

And while semen isn't the most delicious thing in the world, it certainly doesn't taste bad. It's about a teaspoon's worth of thick, salty liquid that, incidentally, should not be confused with urine. It's physically impossible for a man to piss when he's got an erection.

Once you're familiar with the taste and feel of a man's come, swallowing it becomes a natural part of oral sex. Most women really enjoy it. And swallowing semen can't make you pregnant.

A man can also use his mouth to stimulate a woman's genitals. And oral sex is a good way to bring a woman to orgasm, especially if she has trouble reaching orgasm when she's fucking.

Women respond quickly to oral sex because the clitoris is stimulated directly by the tongue. But the clitoris isn't the only part of a woman's genitals.

It feels good if the man licks and kisses the whole area of the vulva, running his tongue from the clitoris down to the vaginal opening, and back up again. Or if he pushes his tongue in and out of the vagina, stimulating the sensitive skin around the entrance.

Stroking the woman's breasts or buttocks will increase her excitement. And if you put a finger inside the vagina while you're licking and kissing, it will give a woman even more intense pleasure.

As the pleasure builds, you can concentrate more on exciting the clitoris, rubbing it harder with your tongue as the woman is reaching orgasm.

And when she comes, the woman will want the stimulation to continue—the same way a man wants his penis sucked all during his orgasm. But when orgasm is over, the clitoris may be very sensitive, so the man should caress the woman's genitals very gently.

A man and woman can take turns stimulating each other with their mouths, or they can do it together at the same time. If you lie on your sides or on top of each other, you can both put your mouth on each other's genitals.

Giving head to each other at the same time—which is called 69—can be twice as much fun. It feels good in your mouth as well as your genitals. You're getting sexual pleasure in your own body, and you also get the excitement that comes from giving your partner pleasure.

And 69 is a very intimate way of having sex. Your mouth, your hands, your genitals, your whole body is in contact with your partner. You can kiss, stroke, taste, and feel each other all at the same time.

Oral sex is a good way to make it when you don't have any birth control. But it's not just a substitute for intercourse.

It's a very pleasurable way to share your body, and that's the best reason for it.

ANAL SEX

Although nobody talks about it very much, the ass is also a very sensitive part of the body. The anus is a tight muscle that's richly supplied with erotic nerves. And just as the mouth can be used for more than eating food, the ass can be used for more than eliminating it. In fact, using the ass for sexual pleasure is fairly common among both men and women.

Most people who haven't tried anal sex assume that the anus is dirty. It can be, just like your ears or your mouth can be dirty if you don't wash them. But the shit is stored several inches up inside the intestines, and if you've washed, the anus itself should be as clean as any other opening to your body.

The anus is connected with the genitals in several important ways. During orgasm a man's anus will always contract in spasms along with his penis. Sometimes women have contractions in their anus too, just like the vagina.

Several inches up inside a man's ass the rectum touches the back of the sensitive prostate gland. This gland produces some of the fluid that goes into a man's ejaculation, and at the point of orgasm it contracts to squeeze the liquid through a series of tubes and out the penis.

A man can always be made to come by inserting a finger into his ass and massaging the prostate gland. If a man is having difficulty reaching orgasm, this can be as effective for him as touching the clitoris is for a woman.

But inserting a finger into the anus should be done gently and gradually. Putting a bit of your own saliva or the natural lubrication from your genitals on your finger will cut down the discomfort and increase the pleasure.

The anus is very similar to the vagina in many ways. And anal intercourse—using the ass for fucking—is something that men and women discovered a long time ago. A lot of couples try it at one time or another, just for fun or curiosity.

The average penis, however, is not going to fit into the average anus without a certain amount of coaxing. It's a tight fit. And doing it for the first time can be as difficult for a woman as losing her virginity.

First you definitely need some kind of lubrication like vaseline. The man should apply this lubricant generously to the woman's anus and to the head of his penis. If the man inserts his finger into the woman's ass, it will help spread the lubricant around, and a gentle fucking motion with the finger will help relax the anal muscle.

The easiest way to have anal intercourse is for the woman to bend forward on her hands and knees. If the man holds his penis against the anus, the woman can push back at her own speed. Several small in-and-out movements are probably better than one deep thrust.

Once the penis is inside, stop for a moment so the woman can adjust to the new sensations. It's best if the woman tries to relax her anal muscle as much as possible, pushing her bowels out rather than squeezing them together.

For a man anal intercourse feels very much like regular fucking. For a woman it can provide unique erotic sensations—but it can also provide a certain amount of discomfort.

To increase the woman's pleasure the man should use his hands to caress the rest of the woman's body, especially her clitoris. The more sexually excited a woman is, the more she can enjoy anal sex. And if the man can hold back his orgasm until the woman is ready, you can both come at the same time.

After anal intercourse a woman's ass is liable to feel sore for a while. That's normal. You haven't damaged anything, it's just that your ass isn't used to it. With practice a woman can learn to relax her anal muscle so it won't hurt.

Just one precaution—if a man inserts his fingers or his penis into a woman's anus, he should not put them into the vagina without washing first. The anus has natural bacteria, just like the mouth, which are harmless and healthy in their proper place. But if these tiny organisms are transferred to the vagina, they can cause minor vaginal infections. So use soap and water before moving from the ass to the vagina.

Touching and stroking each other's ass is a normal part of male-female sex. And whether you go in for anal intercourse or not, there's nothing wrong with it. It's just another way of exploring and enjoying your entire body.

DOING WHAT COMES NATURALLY

Having sex may sound technical and complicated at times. But it's really not. It's a natural instinct, and you know that from your own body. The best way to have sex is simply to do what feels good.

Sex isn't just a matter of position or technique. It's a matter of enjoying your body and enjoying your partner's body. Knowing how to touch and stimulate each other is important, but it's something you have to learn as you go along.

There are lots of ways to have sex. And anything a man and woman do to give each other pleasure is perfectly healthy. That includes using your hands, your mouth, your ass, your genitals, and anything else that appeals to you.

8

SEXUAL IDENTITY

Everybody is born either male or female. But that doesn't say much except what our genitals look like and what society will expect of us.

Just being born a male or female doesn't say what our sexual identity will be when we grow up. It doesn't say whether we'll be attracted to our own sex, the opposite sex, or both sexes.

Most of us turn out to be heterosexuals—that is, we're primarily attracted to the opposite sex. This may be partly a matter of instinct, but it also has a lot to do with social conditioning. From the day we're born we're taught what our sexual role should be by parents, schools, and society.

According to society, men and women are supposed to be sexual opposites. Males are taught to be strong and aggressive toward women. Females are taught to be soft and rather passive toward men. And then, according to the script, men and women are supposed to fall in love, get married, and use their sex to produce more kids.

But it doesn't always work out that simply. Some people find they're attracted to their own sex, and other people dig both sexes. Nobody seems to worry about getting married, and there are lots of reasons for having sex besides reproduction.

Human sexuality is very flexible. And if we grew up alone on a desert island, we would probably have the capacity to respond sexually to both men and women.

But we grow up in a society that attempts to control our sexual behavior by calling one kind of sex "normal" and another kind of sex "queer." Everything we're taught is designed to make us heterosexuals and to make us afraid of sexual contact with our own sex. Men especially are encouraged to avoid intimacy with other men and to ridicule homosexuals.

Nevertheless, homosexuality seems to be a universal human reality. It's found in all societies, in all periods of history. Even animals have homosexual relations. And despite society's prohibitions, a surprisingly high percentage of ordinary men and women have had some kind of sexual experience with their own sex.

All kids, for example, go through a period just before puberty when they hate the opposite sex and get crushes on friends or older members of their own sex. That's a normal part of everybody's sexual development.

Many people's first sexual experience is with somebody of the same sex. It's easier for many kids to explore their sexual curiosity with a friend than to approach a member of the opposite sex.

And some people have occasional homosexual experiences all their lives. And yet most of these people are straight heterosexuals who love and enjoy the opposite sex.

According to a lot of scientific studies like the Kinsey Report, nearly half of all men and one-third of all women admit to being sexually attracted to a member of their own sex at one time or another.

And almost a quarter of all the people in this country have had a real sexual experience to the point of orgasm with a member of their own sex.

Does this mean that everybody is a homosexual? No, but it does mean that many people are capable of enjoying sex with both men and women, and that a certain amount of sexual experimentation is perfectly normal.

There's a lot of difference between having a few homosexual experiences and deciding to be exclusively homosexual all your life. One or two experiences never changed a person's basic sexual identity—after all, there are plenty of homosexuals who have had a few experiences with the opposite sex too.

Some people think that if they have a homosexual dream that means they're going to be homosexual. That's nonsense—everybody has dreams about their own sex, just like everybody has dreams about the opposite sex.

Nobody really knows what makes one person heterosexual and another person homosexual. It doesn't seem to be a matter of body chemistry, and it doesn't depend on whether you like or dislike the opposite sex. Many people think sexual identity depends on how you're brought up, and that a kid with a strong mother and a weak father will become homosexual. But that explanation has been proved false over and over again.

Sexual identity seems to be largely a matter of instinct—it depends on how you feel about yourself and what kind of sex appeals to you.

Everybody has to find their own sexual identity, just like they have to discover the rest of their personality. And it often involves exploring and experimenting. Most sexual experimentation occurs with the opposite sex, but if some of it happens with your own sex, it's not going to hurt you.

Homosexuality isn't some kind of superaddictive drug that once you try it you'll be hooked for life. And being heterosexual isn't like living in a straitjacket. You can experiment with other kinds of sex without losing your sexual identity. The point is not to be worried or frightened about sex—any kind of sex.

HOMOSEXUALITY

Homosexuals are people who prefer making it with somebody of their own sex—men who are sexually attracted to men, women who are sexually attracted to other women.

Homosexuals are not a different race of human beings; they just have a different sexual identity. At least 10 million people in this country consider themselves homosexual, and there is as much diversity and variety among them as among heterosexuals. All kinds of people from bankers to rock stars are attracted to their own sex. Some are conservative and secretive about their sexual identity. Others, especially young homosexuals, are proud of their sexuality and openly identify themselves as gay.

Social stereotypes, though, make it seem like all homosexual men have limp wrists and high voices. And homosexual women—called lesbians—are all supposed to get crew cuts and wear men's clothing. That's a myth.

There are some homosexuals who imitate the dress and mannerisms of the opposite sex, but they're a minority. The vast majority of homosexual men and women are indistinguishable from the rest of society. Homosexual men don't have to be any less masculine, and lesbians don't have to be any less feminine than heterosexuals. There are homosexual men who are construction workers and homosexual women who are fashion models.

And being homosexual doesn't mean automatically disliking the opposite sex. In fact, many homosexual men and women have had a lot of experience with the opposite sex before they discovered their homosexuality. And some homosexuals continue to make it with the opposite sex from time to time all their lives, just like many heterosexuals have occasional homosexual relations.

In bed homosexuals do pretty much the same things that heterosexuals do. Lesbians have oral sex or bring each other to orgasm with their hands. Male homosexuals stimulate each other's genitals with their hands and mouths, or they have anal intercourse.

And homosexuals have as many different kinds of relationships as anybody else. They have sex for fun, for curiosity, or for love. Some homosexuals go through many different partners, and others form a lasting relationship with one person and live together like a married couple.

Many people think that homosexuals all lead miserable,

unhappy lives. That's not true. There are plenty of happy, healthy homosexuals. Homosexuals do have a lot of problems, but most of the problems aren't caused by sex, they're caused by society.

Our society, of course, prohibits homosexuality. Making it with your own sex is considered a crime, a sin, a perversion, or a sickness. And homosexuals have been ridiculed and discriminated against just for enjoying their own bodies.

Homosexuality is illegal, even for consenting adults in the privacy of their own home, in almost every state of this country. Sodomy, as homosexual relations are legally called, is usually defined as some kind of "crime against nature." You'd think homosexuals were polluting the air and water like big corporations.

In this country homosexuals can't work for the government, and no homosexual from another country can become a citizen. If a person is discovered to be gay, he can be thrown out of the army, lose his job, or even be denied a driver's license. So many people have kept their homosexuality a secret in order to avoid being harassed. Although society condemns all homosexuality, men are persecuted more than women. Tens of thousands of men have been arrested and sent to jail for being homosexual, but no woman has ever been locked up for being a lesbian.

Men are probably victimized more than women because the laws are made and enforced by other men. Legislators, policemen, and judges are more uptight about male homosexuality than they are about female homosexuality.

One of the arguments used to persecute homosexuals is the need "to protect society." It's a common belief, for example, that homosexuals are child molesters—people who sexually attack young kids. But it's been shown that the vast majority of child molesters are, in fact, heterosexuals.

Nevertheless, our society considers homosexuality a sickness. Doctors and psychiatrists have usually treated homosexuality as some kind of mental illness that has to be cured. But shrinks have been remarkably unsuccessful in changing anybody's basic sexual orientation. Gay people spend years in therapy and still prefer their own sex. And doctors have devised absolutely inhuman "cures" like giving homosexuals electric shocks and cutting out part of their brain to make them conform to the rest of society. But even these methods don't work.

What society overlooks in all of these prescriptions is that most homosexuals don't want to be cured. They enjoy their own sexuality with people they're sexually attracted to. What most homosexuals need in order to live happier lives is not a change in their sexual identity but a change in society's attitudes.

In many other societies homosexuality is an accepted and natural part of the whole sexual spectrum. And in countries where it isn't encouraged it is at least tolerated. But in the United States we have the harshest laws against homosexuals and the greatest amount of social persecution of any society in the world. That probably says more about how sexually uptight our society is than it says about homosexuality.

BISEXUALITY

Our society likes to put everybody in neat little categories. It likes to think that people are either completely heterosexual or completely homosexual. But there are many people whose sexual identity doesn't fit into either one of these simple extremes.

People who have sex with both men and women are usually called bisexual. But the term bisexual is used so loosely that it can mean just about anything.

Sexual identity is largely a matter of how you see yourself. And most people consider themselves either heterosexual or homosexual regardless of a few sexual experiences that may be different.

The real bisexual is someone who is equally attracted to both sexes and who actively seeks both male and female sex partners. Genuine bisexuals seem to be less common than homosexuals, probably because there are too many problems of sexual identity involved in going back and forth from one sex to the other.

Aside from their unconventional sexual preferences, it would be difficult to identify bisexuals. Bisexuals aren't physically different from anybody else, and there's no special bisexual personality or behavior. Probably you wouldn't know if somebody was bisexual unless he told you.

And bisexuals are not a single group, there are many different kinds of people who are attracted to both sexes. Some bisexuals are married and occasionally make it with a member of their own sex on the side. Other bisexuals have a homosexual lover for a while and then take a lover of the opposite sex. And there are some people with a free sexual life-style who make it equally with men and women all the time.

But having one or two sexual experiences with either sex doesn't make a person bisexual. Usually it takes several years of both homosexual and heterosexual experience before people decide they're really bisexual. And it all depends on whether or not you want to be a bisexual, whether you're attracted to both sexes, and how you feel about your own sexual identity.

SEXUAL ROLES

Sexual roles are beginning to change for everybody in our society—for men and women, heterosexuals and homosexuals.

The old stereotypes for the ideal man and woman are breaking down. Young people are working out their own definitions of what's masculine and what's feminine. Women are discovering that brains and beauty aren't mutually exclusive and men are finding out they have emotions as well as muscles.

Men and women are a lot more equal today than they were twenty years ago. This is a result of lots of things, like birth control, the sexual revolution, and the women's liberation movement. The result is that heterosexuals are finding new ways of relating to each other as sexual partners, without getting hung up on machismo or marriage.

Homosexuals are also rejecting the stereotypes society has created for them. The gay liberation movement is encouraging homosexual men and women to come out in the open and express themselves—not only as homosexuals but also as human beings.

After all, there's more to people than their sexual preference. Nobody spends their entire life in bed. And expecting everybody to live up to a sexual stereotype just prevents people from developing their individuality.

The trouble with sexual stereotypes is that they're never true. Most men and women just don't look or live like the people in movies.

Sexual roles are a matter of what you want for yourself. Some people find their sexual role easily and naturally, for others it involves searching and experimenting.

But the sexual revolution of the last ten years has made it possible for people to explore their sexual personalities. And when people are free to experiment, they can base their sexual choices on what they like instead of what they're afraid of. Fear of the opposite sex isn't a good reason for being homosexual, and fear of homosexuals isn't a sensible reason for being heterosexual.

Heterosexuals, homosexuals, and bisexuals aren't three different kinds of people. They're all basically the same people—it's just that they've found three different ways to express and enjoy their sexuality.

And today young people are finding that they have more in common with each other, whether they're male or female, heterosexual or homosexual, than they have in common with their parents' generation.

9

PREGNANCY

Reproduction is the one area of sex we're liable to be told something about—if our parents or schools tell us anything at all.

But most parents aren't too clear on the subject themselves. And the way sex is taught in school, plants and people and fish usually get lumped together in one breath. Learning about human reproduction often consists of little more than memorizing long lists of technical terms that don't mean anything.

All this can make pregnancy seem remote and unreal—as though it didn't have anything to do with sex.

But pregnancy—especially the danger of an unwanted pregnancy—is a real fact of life for anyone who's having sex. A lot of women under the age of eighteen get pregnant by accident, and most of these accidents happen because young men and women aren't given the kind of information they need to protect themselves.

Knowing how your reproductive organs work has some very

practical benefits. It makes it easier to understand what's happening in your own body from day to day and from month to month. It enables you to recognize the symptoms of pregnancy early, while there's still time to get help. But most of all, knowing something about reproduction makes it easier to understand birth control and how to use it.

REPRODUCTIVE ORGANS

Pregnancy starts when a sperm cell finds its way through a woman's reproductive organs and fertilizes an egg.

That sounds simple enough, but the whole process of fertilization and pregnancy is far more complicated. It doesn't begin with the penis and vagina, but with the testicles and the ovaries.

A man's testicles and a woman's ovaries perform two major jobs. First, they produce hormones that regulate sexual growth and functioning all our lives. Second, they manufacture the sperm and egg that are needed for reproduction.

A man's testicles produce the male sex hormone called testosterone. A woman's ovaries produce the female hormones, estrogen and progesterone. It's these hormones that shape and control our sexuality.

During puberty large amounts of these hormones are pumped into the bloodstream, causing the body to sexually mature. This stage of sexual development usually begins around the age of ten in females and a year or so later in males. During the next several years the genitals grow in size, body hair begins to sprout, women develop breasts, and the internal reproductive organs begin to function.

A girl knows her reproductive system is starting to work when she begins to menstruate. The first period signals the beginning of fertility.

The male counterpart to this is ejaculation. During childhood a boy can have erections and even orgasms, but nothing comes out of the penis. The first ejaculation of semen means that his body is getting ready for reproduction.

But the early menstrual periods and the early ejaculations

don't necessarily mean that the body is completely fertile yet. During puberty a man's testicles may not produce much sperm, and a woman's ovaries may produce eggs only sporadically.

The reproductive organs actually need time to warm up, and it may take several years before a person is fully capable of reproducing. When the internal organs are mature, the testicles produce sperm continuously and the ovaries produce eggs on a regular cycle.

The sperm and the egg are the two halves of human reproduction. Together they start a pregnancy.

Sperm cells are being manufactured all the time inside a man's testicles. But to reach the outside world they have to travel through a long series of tubes inside a man's body for several weeks. This journey gives the sperm the time they need to mature.

As the sperm leave the testicles, they first pass through long, coiled tubes that sit on top of each testicle. Then the sperm travel up two straight tubes until they reach the seminal vesicles—two ducts where the sperm is stored until it is ready to be ejaculated.

The seminal vesicles also produce part of the fluid that makes up a man's semen. It's this fluid that carries the sperm out of the penis during ejaculation.

When ejaculation starts, the seminal vesicles contract, forcing the sperm and liquid into the urethra. The prostate gland also contracts and squeezes its own fluid into the urethra. The liquids and sperm mix together as they travel down the urethra and come out of the penis as semen in four or five spurts.

Although there are about 400 million sperm cells in the average ejaculation, sperm is just a small portion of the semen. The bulk of semen consists of fluids from the seminal vesicles and the prostate gland. In fact, the microscopic sperm cells are so small that you couldn't see the difference in the amount of semen if all 400 million sperm were removed.

Since the testicles are constantly producing new sperm, there's no possibility of using it all up. If a man comes a few times in the same day, the amount of sperm will be slightly reduced, but there will still be many millions of sperm cells in each ejaculation. This means that once a man reaches sexual maturity he's capable of reproducing all the time.

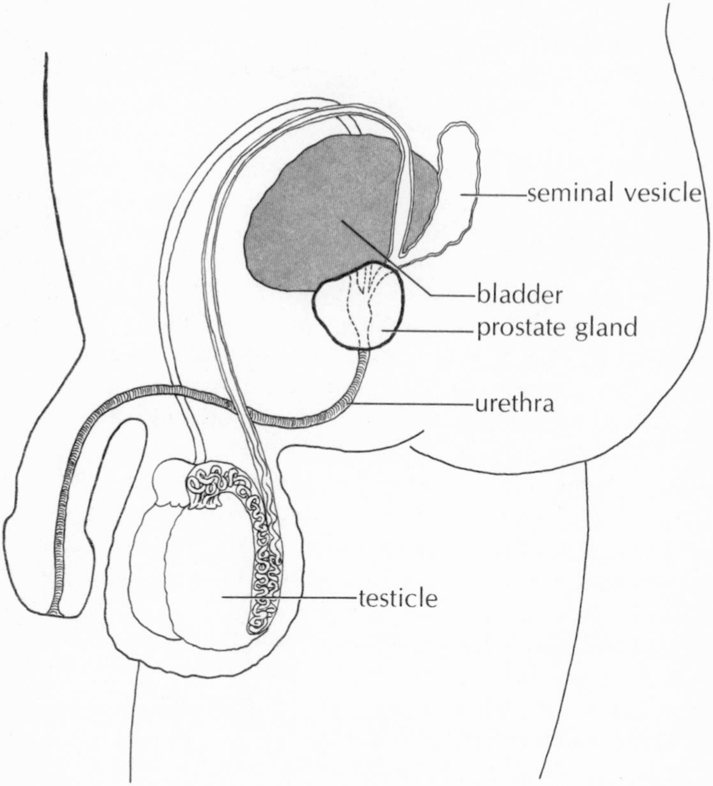

THE MALE REPRODUCTIVE SYSTEM: sperm travels from the testicles, through a series of tubes, before being ejaculated from the penis.

In fact, this constant production of sperm is one reason why a man physically needs to have sex. As the two seminal vesicles get filled with sperm, they create a need for sexual release. If a man doesn't have an orgasm for a week or two, the seminal vesicles will naturally empty themselves through a wet dream in order to make room for new sperm.

For a man sexual pleasure and reproduction are really the same process. A man needs sexual pleasure in order to release his sperm.

A woman's body is different in this respect. Her reproductive system functions independent of sexual pleasure—she doesn't need an orgasm to get pregnant.

A woman's ovaries are located in the lower abdomen. Two fallopian tubes lead from the ovaries into the uterus, and the mouth of the uterus—called the cervix—opens into the vagina. These are the basic parts of the female reproductive system.

A woman is born with all her eggs already inside the ovaries. In fact, each ovary contains hundreds of thousands of immature eggs. These eggs are slightly bigger than sperm cells, but even so, they're barely visible to the naked eye.

When a woman's reproductive organs are mature, the ovaries take turns releasing a single ripened egg each month. This process, known as ovulation, usually takes place about two weeks before a woman gets her period.

When an egg is released from the ovary, it passes into a fallopian tube. For several days it travels down the fallopian tube toward the uterus. If no sperm are present to fertilize the egg while it's still in the fallopian tube, the egg will simply die.

The uterus, meanwhile, has been preparing itself in case fertilization should occur. The walls of the uterus have been building up a thick lining in which the fertilized egg can bury itself and start to grow.

But if the egg hasn't been fertilized, the lining isn't needed. In that case, the lining breaks away from the uterine walls. Together with the unused egg and a few ounces of blood, it flows through the cervix, down through the vagina, and out of the body.

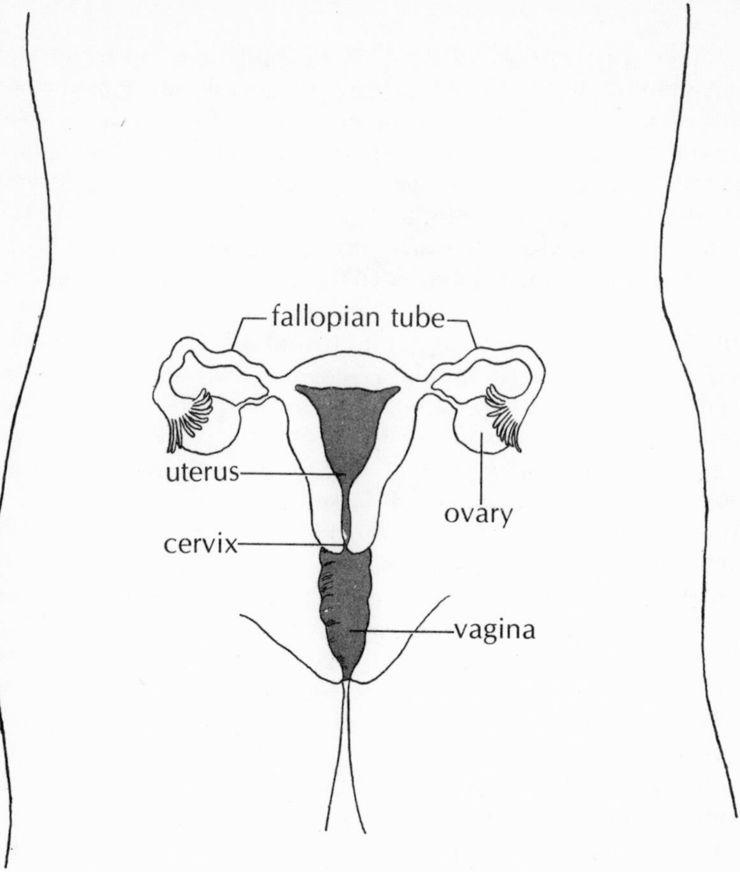

THE FEMALE REPRODUCTIVE SYSTEM: egg travels from an ovary, through a fallopian tube, into the uterus.

This is the monthly process of menstruation. And although menstruation is usually thought of as the end of a reproductive cycle, it's also the beginning of a new one.

As a woman is shedding the uterine lining, another egg is maturing inside one of her ovaries. The new egg will be released, and the uterus will build another lining, which will be shed again if no pregnancy occurs.

The average menstrual cycle is 28 days long—counting from the first day of one period to the first day of the next period. But 28 days is just an average, and many women have menstrual cycles considerably longer or shorter than average.

For example, when a woman first starts menstruating, her periods are often irregular. It takes several years for the body to establish a regular cycle, and a young woman's periods may come three weeks apart sometimes and five weeks apart at other times. She may even skip a period altogether. Variations like these are all perfectly normal.

Even mature women don't necessarily have 28-day menstrual cycles. Some women have regular cycles of 20 days, others menstruate every 40 days. And there are many women whose cycle is never regular at all.

The menstrual routine is easily influenced by a variety of psychological, physical, and emotional factors. If a woman is especially nervous one month, her period may be delayed, or it may come sooner than she expected.

Traveling, fatigue, excitement, tension, and dieting can have unpredictable effects on menstruation. Students, for example, often miss a period during exam time. And if a woman is worried about being pregnant, her anxiety may, in fact, delay the period.

But the reproductive system in both men and women functions the same way whether or not you're having sex. In other words, a man will constantly produce and store sperm. If he's not having sex, he'll ejaculate the sperm anyway through wet dreams.

And a woman will release an egg each month, build a thick uterine lining in preparation for pregnancy, and have menstrual periods even if she's a virgin.

GETTING PREGNANT

When a man ejaculates inside a woman's vagina during intercourse, millions of sperm are released in his semen. These sperm swim blindly around the vagina, up through the cervix, around the walls of the uterus, and into the fallopian tubes.

If there's a mature egg waiting in one of the fallopian tubes, the sperm can fertilize it and start a pregnancy.

Most of the sperm die before they can reach the egg, and it's possible they could all die on their journey. But it takes only one successful sperm cell to fertilize an egg.

The egg that is released from a woman's ovary usually doesn't live much longer than twenty-four hours. This means that a woman can get pregnant only on the day or two following ovulation. But the problem here is that it's almost impossible for most women to tell exactly when they ovulate.

Ovulation is supposed to take place about two weeks before a woman is due to get her next period. But the menstrual cycle can vary a great deal, and young women are especially irregular when it comes to ovulation. They may not ovulate at all for the first several years of menstruation, or they may ovulate sporadically and at unpredictable times during each menstrual cycle.

It's also impossible to tell how long sperm may live inside a woman's reproductive system. Sperm cells usually die in a day or two, but they've been known to survive for as long as a week.

This means that it's possible for a woman to get pregnant several days after she has had intercourse—provided the sperm stay alive inside her fallopian tubes until an egg is released.

As soon as one sperm cell penetrates the egg, a pregnancy has begun. The fertilized egg immediately forms a hard shell to prevent any other sperm from entering. Then it continues down the fallopian tube and into the uterus.

Here it sticks to the thick lining on the wall of the uterus and begins to grow. The pregnant woman will stop having menstrual periods because the uterine lining is now needed to nourish the developing fetus.

The whole process of pregnancy normally takes about nine

months. But the fetus doesn't begin to physically resemble a human being until the third month, and it usually cannot survive outside the woman's body until the seventh month.

When the baby is ready to be born, muscular contractions in the woman's body will force it out of the uterus, through the vagina, and into the outside world.

Like any other part of the body, the reproductive system can occasionally malfunction. Every now and then an egg gets fertilized while it's still in the ovary, or a fertilized egg can get stuck in the fallopian tube. These accidents of nature can cause very serious medical problems.

But for most of us the real concern at the moment is not how to have a successful pregnancy but how to tell if you're pregnant and what to do about it.

HOW TO TELL IF YOU'RE PREGNANT

Most women first suspect they may be pregnant when their period doesn't come on time.

Missing a period can simply be the result of dieting, tension, or fatigue. But of course it can also be the result of pregnancy.

There are several other physical signs that a woman might notice. Morning sickness is common during the first three months of pregnancy. And a woman's breasts may enlarge or feel especially sensitive.

But these changes can be so slight that a woman may not associate them with pregnancy. And there are many women who don't experience these early signs at all.

So if your period is late—two weeks late—it's important to find out quickly whether or not you're pregnant by getting a pregnancy test.

A pregnancy test is a very simple procedure. A sample of your urine is analyzed to see if it contains a certain hormone that is found only during pregnancy. If the test results are positive, it means the hormone is present and you're pregnant. If the test results are negative, it means the hormone is not present and you're not pregnant.

It's important to remember, however, that pregnancy tests

are not 100 percent accurate during the first few weeks of pregnancy. The hormone in question can be present in a woman's urine as early as the third week, but there may not be enough of it to show up until a woman is four or five weeks pregnant.

So it's possible to get a false negative even though you're several weeks pregnant. This doesn't happen very often, but it's good to keep in mind. If your test is negative, and your period still hasn't come after a few weeks, return to the doctor and have a second pregnancy test. The second time the results will be more reliable.

Of all the medical help a sexually active woman may need during her life, a pregnancy test is probably the least hassle. It's quick, painless, and usually very cheap. Many clinics will simply ask you to drop off a sample of your urine and then phone the next day for the results.

If your pregnancy test is done by a private doctor, he may also give you a pelvic examination to double-check the results of the urine analysis. During the pelvic exam he'll check the vagina, the cervix, and the uterus by inserting a gloved finger into your vagina and feeling the internal organs. This examination may be awkward, but it doesn't hurt.

It's natural to want to avoid seeing a doctor, but don't trust any of the do-it-yourself pregnancy testing kits now on the market. These kits do not work—they simply don't produce accurate results. Your urine sample must be analyzed by a medical laboratory.

It's also natural to panic when you think you're pregnant and put off the pregnancy test in the hope that your period will come if you just give it a little more time. But delay can only cause trouble.

If you are pregnant, you'll need the time to figure out what you're going to do. And if you're not pregnant, you'll only be putting yourself through weeks of unnecessary anxiety.

WHERE TO GET A PREGNANCY TEST

Getting a pregnancy test without your parents' knowledge or permission is pretty easy in most big cities. In fact, you can usually take your choice among a variety of private and public services.

But it's important to keep in mind that an unmarried woman under the age of eighteen is still a minor, and in many states there are restrictions on what medical care, if any, a minor can get without parental consent.

In some states specific laws enable any minor to give her own consent for a pregnancy test. In other states there are minimum-age requirements or conditions like being married or "emancipated"—that is, self-supporting and living away from home. In some states the laws are so absurd that they say you have to be pregnant before you can get a pregnancy test.

Health laws vary a great deal from state to state. In fact, they're so confusing and contradictory that doctors and clinics often ignore them, especially when it comes to a simple pregnancy test.

In California, for example, the law says that a minor must be married, pregnant, or emancipated before she can get medical care on her own. But you can get a pregnancy test almost anywhere in California, regardless of age, with no hassle at all.

In New York the law stipulates that minors under eighteen must be married or have a child in order to give their own medical consent. But these conditions are routinely overlooked, even by the Public Health Department. And it's easy for any minor to get a pregnancy test on her own, especially in the large cities.

In many states the law makes no provision for minors getting their own medical care. But this still doesn't mean you can't get a confidential pregnancy test. There are many exceptions for "emergency" treatment, and doctors are allowed a wide range of discretion. All it means is that you may run into a private doctor who refuses to treat you. In that case, try another doctor or clinic.

If you think you're going to have a hassle with any doctor or clinic, you can always lie about your name, your age, your marital status, or your independence. As long as you pay the bill, nobody will ever know or care.

Hawaii is about the only state where the law might present a real problem. The law there says that any female between the ages of fourteen and eighteen can give her own consent for a pregnancy test, but if the test comes out positive, the doctor is required to inform her parents. This means that in Hawaii you'll have to phone around to find a friendly doctor or clinic that ignores the law.

In fact, it's a good idea to phone any service in any state to check it out first. If you want to avoid private doctors altogether, there are many other private and public services you can call. Ask if they give confidential pregnancy tests to a woman your age. Somewhere along the line you'll be able to find a cheap, reliable service without having to involve your parents if you don't want to.

Private doctors. All general practitioners can give pregnancy tests. So can gynecologists—doctors who specialize in women's health care.

Every doctor in your city will be listed in the yellow pages under "Physicians." Chances are, you'll want to avoid your family doctor, since he'll know your parents.

There are two drawbacks to seeing a private doctor. First, they're expensive. Doctors' fees range from $10 to $25 and higher.

The second drawback is that private doctors, especially gynecologists, often have a long waiting list for appointments. But if you think you're pregnant, you can't afford to wait two or three weeks. Explain that you want a pregnancy test, or insist that your case is an emergency. If you can't get an appointment quickly, try another doctor or another service.

Public health departments. In most cities the public health department runs a number of services like neighborhood clinics and public hospitals that give pregnancy tests. The cost will be minimal. You can find the telephone number for your local health department in the phone book, and ask about their pregnancy testing services.

Hospitals. All hospitals do pregnancy tests, but they may require parental permission. Call your local hospital and ask them for specific information about pregnancy tests. Public hospitals often have special family planning or maternity clinics that offer inexpensive pregnancy tests.

Planned Parenthood. Planned Parenthood is a national organization with nearly 200 centers across the country. Although their primary service is to provide birth control, most of their centers also give pregnancy tests. If your local Planned Parenthood doesn't give pregnancy tests, it will probably be able to refer you to a place that does. Planned Parenthood is inexpensive, and their staff is generally sympathetic.

Free clinics. Free clinics are not necessarily free, but they all serve young people. They're usually very inexpensive and staffed by sympathetic young doctors. Free clinics in your area may advertise in local underground newspapers, or they may be listed in the yellow pages under "Clinics."

Women's health centers. Women's groups have set up small health centers in many large cities during the last few years. These centers frequently offer a wide range of services to women in need of medical help. Many of them give pregnancy tests, and those that don't can usually refer you to another service that does.

Like free clinics, women's health centers in your area may advertise in local underground newspapers, or they may be listed in the yellow pages under "Clinics."

Clergy consultation service on abortion. The Clergy Consultation Service is a nationwide abortion referral service, but it will also give you information on where to get a pregnancy test. It's a very reliable organization, which is accustomed to helping young women who don't want their parents involved. If your pregnancy test is positive and you want to have an abortion, they will help you arrange it for the lowest possible cost.

Hotlines and switchboards. There are hundreds of telephone hotlines across the country, and many of them answer questions about sex and make referrals for medical services. A hotline in your area will almost always know the best place to go for a pregnancy test.

Some hotlines, free clinics, women's health centers, and public services are listed in the last chapter of this book, as well as all local chapters of Planned Parenthood and the Clergy Consultation Service. Check the list to see what's available in your area.

10

BIRTH CONTROL

Having sex doesn't have to involve getting pregnant. It doesn't even have to involve worrying about pregnancy. There are several convenient, reliable methods of birth control, and all it takes to use them successfully is a little information and planning.

If you want to avoid an accidental pregnancy, you have to use some kind of birth control every time you have intercourse. A woman is never completely safe from pregnancy—not even during her period.

And that means sex will always require a little planning.

It's nice to think of sex as a spontaneous act of passion, but it's not realistic. Sex is never completely spontaneous, it always involves making some kind of decisions. And choosing a method of birth control is the first decision you should make.

Getting the right birth-control device is not something you can leave to the last minute. And it's not something you should assume your partner will take care of. Especially if you haven't discussed the problem together.

Sometimes people are embarrassed about getting birth control. Or they may feel shy about using it. But risking an unwanted pregnancy to avoid a few uncomfortable moments doesn't make much sense. And although birth control might be a hassle at first, it soon becomes a routine part of your sex life.

Society has tried to make it difficult for young people to get birth-control information and devices in order to keep you from fucking. But it should be obvious to everybody that this tactic doesn't work.

Forty percent of all illegitimate babies are born to teenage mothers, and one-third of the women who marry before the age of eighteen are already pregnant.

The effort of parents and schools to prevent young people from using birth control has resulted only in disrupted lives, forced marriages, unwanted babies, unnecessary abortions, and a lot of needless worry.

But you don't have to fall into any of these traps. And you don't have to rely on home remedies and methods that won't work. Reliable birth-control devices are available, and despite society's obstacles, you can get them if you want.

These devices fall into five categories: condoms, spermicides, diaphragms, intrauterine devices, and birth-control pills. The rest of this chapter will tell you how they work and where you can get them.

CONDOMS

A condom is the only kind of birth-control device that's made for men. It's a thin tube that fits over the entire penis.

Condoms—called rubbers or prophylactics—come in several different varieties. The ordinary condom is made of latex rubber, but more expensive types have special features. For example, some condoms are made from animal skin, some are lubricated, and some have a little tip on the end that acts as a reservoir for the man's semen.

But they all act in the same way to prevent pregnancy. When

a man ejaculates, his semen is trapped inside the condom and never touches the woman's vagina at all. And no sperm get free to start a pregnancy.

Condoms, however, are not foolproof. They can break and they can slip off the penis during intercourse.

So to avoid accidents that can cause pregnancy, condoms have to be handled very carefully. And there are several things a man should always keep in mind when using them.

First, put the condom on as soon as the penis is erect. You shouldn't begin to fuck or even rub the penis against the opening of the vagina before the condom has been put on. The few drops of lubricating fluid that come from a man's cock during sexual excitement often contain enough sperm to make a woman pregnant.

Second, if the condom doesn't have a tip, leave a half inch of space at the end to catch the semen. Otherwise the semen will flow all over the inside of the condom. This can cause it to come loose.

And third, it's important to hold the condom tight against the base of the penis when you withdraw from your partner's vagina. For some reason condoms are always made a little bigger than the average penis, and after orgasm, when your erection starts to go down, it's very easy for the condom to slip off. If this happens, sperm can escape into the woman's vagina.

If condoms are used properly, the chances of avoiding pregnancy are pretty good. But condoms are much safer if the woman also uses a vaginal spermicide. If the condom should accidentally break or come loose, the spermicide will kill any sperm that escape.

Condoms are a very popular method of birth control because they're easy to get. Both men and women can buy them in any drugstore without a prescription, and they're fairly cheap. A package of three costs about $1.50. Some common brands are Trojans, Guardians, Sheiks, and Ramses. If you want them lubricated or with a tip, you have to tell the druggist.

In some states condoms are sold in vending machines in men's rooms. But these may be old, and they're usually poor quality. Drugstore condoms are much more reliable.

A woman who's sexually active can always carry a few condoms in her purse, just in case her partner forgets them. And a man can keep a few condoms in his wallet. But don't carry condoms around for a couple of months, the rubber can get old and break easily.

Besides being cheap and convenient, condoms have other advantages. They're easy to use, they don't interfere with sexual pleasure, and they provide good protection against venereal disease.

SPERMICIDES

Spermicides are a chemical kind of birth control that a woman puts in her vagina before having intercourse. Spermicides prevent pregnancy by killing sperm cells that a man ejaculates into the vagina. And for extra protection they also block the cervix, so that even if some sperm survive, they cannot get through a woman's reproductive system.

Spermicides come in five basic forms: foams, jellies, creams, tablets, and suppositories. The tablets and suppositories are not reliable and should not be used for birth control. The jellies and creams are messy and generally less effective than the foams.

Foam is the best form of spermicide. It coats the inside of the vagina evenly, so it works better than the creams and jellies.

Contraceptive foams come in aerosol cans. When you buy foam for the first time, you must get a kit that includes a plastic applicator and a set of instructions.

The directions should be read thoroughly, but keep in mind that they can be misleading. For example, the directions usually say that foam can be inserted into the vagina up to an hour before intercourse. But it's not a good idea to wait more than a half hour between inserting the foam and having intercourse, since the longer foam stays in the vagina, the less effective it becomes.

To use the foam you fill the applicator from the aerosol can. Then slide the applicator into your vagina as far as it comfortably fits, the same way you insert a tampon. When you push in the plunger, the foam is forced into the vagina. And even though the instructions call for only one applicator of foam, it's safer to use two.

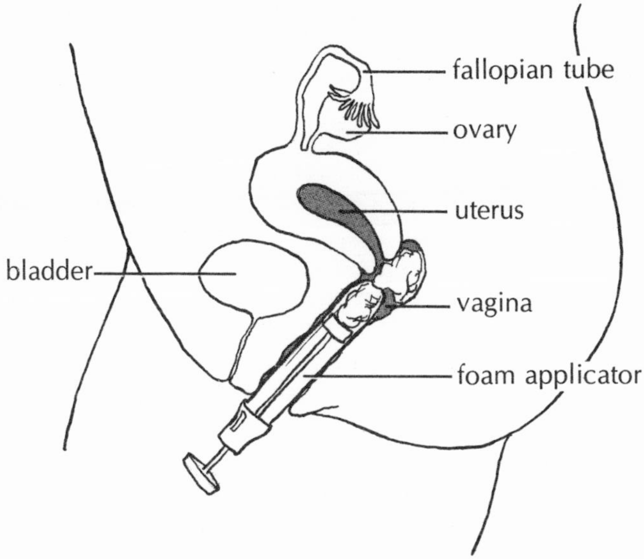

APPLICATOR OF SPERMICIDAL FOAM inserted into vagina

All forms of spermicides melt inside the vagina and are likely to leak out. Although the foam tends to leak less than jellies or creams, you still shouldn't walk around too much after inserting it. If you do, another applicator of foam should be inserted right before intercourse. And you should always put in more foam before having intercourse a second time.

After intercourse you cannot douche for at least six hours, since all that time is needed for the foam to work. You should also avoid taking a bath, because water can enter the vagina and wash out the foam.

Occasionally a man or woman will experience a minor allergic irritation to a particular spermicide. If this happens to you, try a different brand.

The disadvantages of using spermicidal foam for birth control are pretty obvious. You definitely have to plan ahead for intercourse, and inserting foam can be a lot of hassle in certain situations.

But what's more important, contraceptive foams are not completely reliable. In fact, they are the least reliable of the five methods discussed in this chapter. It's possible to get pregnant using foam, even if you follow the directions perfectly.

The best alternative for a woman who does not have any other means of birth control is to use foam while her partner uses a condom. Together the two offer much better birth-control protection.

Despite all these problems, foam has one definite advantage—it's available without prescription in any drugstore. And a kit that includes the applicator costs only about $4. Two common brands are Emko and Delfen.

Whether it's used alone or in combination with condoms, you can't feel the foam inside your vagina, and it doesn't interfere with sexual pleasure. You can even have oral sex without worrying about the foam, since your partner probably won't even notice it.

Foam is completely harmless, it's easy to carry around in your purse, and there's some evidence that it helps protect you against VD.

DIAPHRAGMS

The diaphragm is a shallow rubber cup that fits tightly around the cervix. It's filled with spermicidal jelly and inserted into the vagina before intercourse.

Once it's in place the diaphragm helps to block the opening to the cervix. And any sperm that swim over the rim of the diaphragm are killed by the spermicide.

The diaphragm and jelly must always be used together. One without the other provides only half the protection needed to prevent pregnancy.

The spermicidal jelly can be bought in any drugstore, but you can get the diaphragm only from a doctor or birth-control clinic. Diaphragms come in different sizes, and only a doctor can examine you and determine what size will fit your cervix properly.

So don't be tempted to borrow a diaphragm from a friend—it probably won't fit you right.

A doctor will also teach you how to insert and remove the diaphragm. It's not very difficult to use, but it does require a little practice.

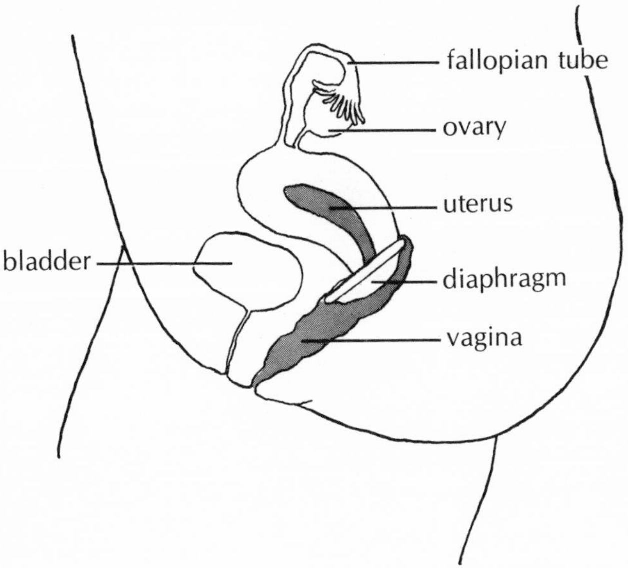

DIAPHRAGM in place over cervix

To insert the diaphragm, you squeeze the rim together, push it into your vagina, then guide it into place over the cervix with a finger.

Removing the diaphragm is easy. You just pull down on the rim and slip it out of the vagina.

Some doctors will give you a plastic device for inserting and removing the diaphragm, but it's better to use your fingers. It's always a good idea to get familiar with the way your vagina feels, and besides, you'll have to put your finger inside your vagina anyway to check that the diaphragm is securely in place.

The doctor should also tell you how to use the jelly. Jelly is usually spread inside the diaphragm before it's inserted, and an applicator full of jelly is put into the vagina after the diaphragm is in place.

Once you get the hang of it, inserting the diaphragm takes only a few seconds. And you can engage in all kinds of physical activity with the diaphragm in place, since it can't be felt and it can't fall out.

You can insert the diaphragm whenever it's convenient, but the jelly is good for only about two hours. So if intercourse is delayed, you'll have to put another applicator of jelly inside your vagina. And more jelly is needed if you have intercourse a second time.

Although the diaphragm looks big, it doesn't interfere with sexual pleasure, and it usually can't be felt by either the man or woman during intercourse. In addition, the diaphragm has the advantage of holding back the menstrual flow if you fuck during your period.

After intercourse the diaphragm and jelly must be left in the vagina for eight hours. The jelly may melt and get a little messy, but you cannot douche during that time. If you have intercourse at night, it usually means that you can't remove the diaphragm or douche until the next day. However, once the initial eight hours are up, it doesn't matter how long the diaphragm stays in place.

Using the diaphragm correctly takes a little discipline. You either have to plan ahead for intercourse or have the willpower to stop when you're making out and insert your diaphragm.

And you can't take any shortcuts with this method of birth control. The jelly must be used each time you have intercourse, and the diaphragm must be left in place a full eight hours afterward.

Although it involves some work, the diaphragm has several benefits. It doesn't produce any physical side effects, it can be used by almost every woman, and it's convenient to carry around in your purse.

A diaphragm is not expensive. It costs only about $5, and it should last about two years. However, you have to consider the cost of a doctor or clinic, and return checkups are necessary once a year to make sure your size hasn't changed.

The jelly is also cheap, it costs about $3 for a large tube. There are a dozen common brands made especially for use with the diaphragm, including Ortho-Gynol Jelly, Lanteen Jelly, and Ramses Jelly. But avoid a product named Koromex, since it contains a dangerously high level of mercury.

There are also spermicidal creams that can be used with a diaphragm, but they usually melt much faster and get messier than jellies. In any case, make sure you get an applicator when you buy jelly or cream for the first time.

Together the diaphragm and jelly offer good protection against pregnancy. When used properly, they're safer than either foams or condoms. And you can use this method of birth control whether you have intercourse regularly or just every once in a while.

INTRAUTERINE DEVICES

An intrauterine device—which is usually called by its initials, IUD—is a small piece of molded plastic or metal that is inserted in the uterus. Scientists don't know exactly how the IUD works, but they do know that once it's inside the uterus a woman is automatically protected from pregnancy.

The IUD comes in a variety of shapes, such as loops, coils, and shields. Some shapes are safer and more effective than others, and in general the plastic IUDs are better than metal ones.

An IUD can be put in place only by a doctor. It's inserted through the vagina, up through the opening in the cervix, and

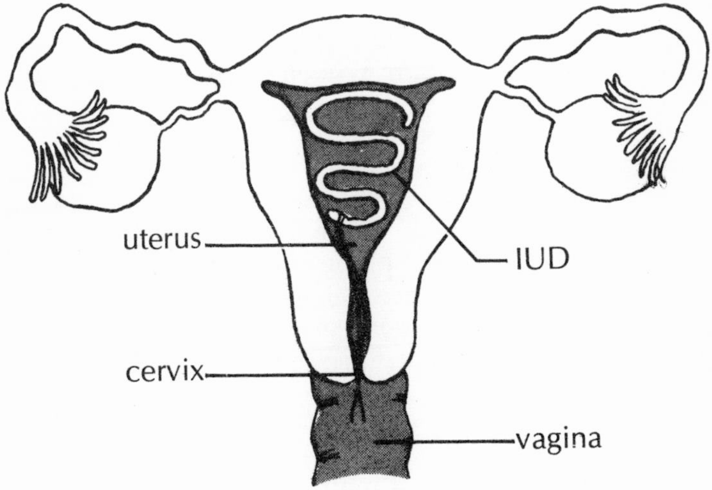

INTRAUTERINE DEVICE (IUD) in place in the uterus

into the uterus. This is usually done during your period, when the cervical opening is wider and insertion is easier.

Once the IUD is in place, it works all by itself without requiring any attention from you. This method is very different from the diaphragm, which has to be inserted and removed every time you have intercourse. The IUD is left inside the uterus indefinitely, providing constant birth-control protection.

A thin nylon string attached to the IUD hangs down into the vagina. You can feel the string by putting a finger inside your vagina, and this will tell you that the device is still there.

If you ever want to have the IUD removed, a doctor can slip it out of your uterus by pulling on the string. But a woman should never try take it out by herself. The cervix may be blocked, or the IUD may get caught, and tugging on the string could be dangerous.

Because the IUD doesn't require any work, it's a very convenient method of birth control. But the IUD can be used safely and successfully by only about 60 to 70 percent of women. And there's no way to tell beforehand whether this device will be safe for you.

Some women experience a lot of pain when the IUD is inserted, and they may have cramps for several days afterward. An IUD can also cause bleeding in between periods and heavy bleeding during menstruation, although these side effects usually disappear after the first few months. Occasionally a woman must have the IUD removed because the cramps are too severe or the bleeding is too heavy.

Some women expel the IUD, because their uterus contracts and pushes the device into the vagina. When this happens, the IUD will simply fall out of the body, and the woman may not even notice it. This presents a real danger, since the woman will continue to have intercourse assuming she's still protected.

And even if the IUD remains properly in place, it still isn't foolproof against pregnancy. Occasionally the IUD will fail to work, and doctors aren't able to tell why or when this will happen.

All these problems occur more frequently to young women and women who have never been pregnant. In fact, many doctors are reluctant to prescribe the IUD for young women. If you want to use this device, you'll have a better chance of getting it from a gynecologist or a birth-control clinic than a general practitioner.

If you are one of the lucky women who can use an IUD without any problems, this method of birth control has several benefits. It's a lot more reliable than condoms, foams, or diaphragms, and it doesn't require any work. You only have to check the string occasionally to see that the device is still in place and return to the doctor at least once a year for a checkup.

You don't have to plan for intercourse, in fact, the IUD doesn't interfere with sex in any way. You can fuck whenever you want, and neither you nor your partner will feel the device.

BIRTH-CONTROL PILLS

Birth-control pills are the most effective kind of contraception available. If you take them as directed, it's practically impossible to get pregnant.

The pills work by imitating the way a woman's body naturally functions during pregnancy. This is what makes them so effective, but it's also what causes their side effects.

When a woman is pregnant, her body produces large amounts of female hormones that prevent her from ovulating until pregnancy is over. Birth-control pills contain synthetic versions of these same hormones, and they produce the same effect. A woman's eggs stay inside her ovaries, where they cannot be fertilized by sperm. As long as a woman takes the pills she won't ovulate at all.

Birth-control pills are powerful medicine, and they have to be prescribed by a doctor or clinic. It's a very dangerous idea to borrow them from a friend or buy them illegally.

Not every woman can safely take birth-control pills. A thorough medical examination by a doctor is the only way to tell if the pills will be safe for you.

And only a doctor can decide which kind of pills are best for your body. There are more than twenty different brands of birth-control pills, and each contains different amounts of the hormones estrogen and progesterone in varying combinations.

Most brands have 21 pills in each pack. Starting on the fifth day of your menstrual cycle, you take one pill every day for three weeks. Then you stop taking the pills for one week so you can have your period.

Some brands have only 20 pills in each pack, and others have 28. The exact schedule for taking these pills is a little different, so it's important to get complete instructions from your doctor.

The effectiveness of birth-control pills depends on keeping a constant supply of hormones in your body. That means you can't just take one pill and be protected, and you can't just take a pill every time you have intercourse. The pills must be taken every day to provide birth-control protection, and a new pack of pills must be started on schedule each month.

Besides preventing ovulation, birth-control pills affect your entire body. And they produce many side effects that are similar to the side effects of early pregnancy.

Nausea, headaches, and depression are common when a woman first starts taking the pills. Some women gain weight, and some women bleed a little in between periods. But these side effects should disappear after a month or two. If they don't, it's important to return to the doctor.

The pills may also enlarge a woman's breasts, and some women report that the pills tend to increase or decrease their sexual appetite. These side effects are not permanent, however, and if you stop taking the pills, your body will return to normal.

The pills also change the natural germ-killing climate inside the vagina, and they make a woman more susceptible to a variety of genital infections.

These side effects are usually minor. The only serious complication caused by birth-control pills is blood clotting. This is very dangerous, but it's also very rare. It happens about as frequently in women who take the pills as it does in women who are pregnant.

Newspapers are always full of scare stories that exaggerate the danger of birth-control pills. But, in fact, women who take the pills are safer than sexually active women who don't. The pill protects you from accidental pregnancy, and many more women die each year from complications of pregnancy and childbirth than from blood clots caused by the pill.

Taking birth-control pills is safer than driving in a car or smoking cigarettes. Although the pills do produce side effects, in the long run they are safer than any other method of birth control available today.

And birth-control pills have other advantages. They automatically produce a regular 28-day menstrual cycle, and they usually reduce the length of your period, the amount of bleeding, and the pain of cramps.

In addition, birth-control pills don't involve planning or preparation for intercourse, and they don't interfere with sexual pleasure in any way. You can have sex whenever you want, including the fourth week of your cycle when no pills are taken.

Birth-control pills are also cheap. A month's supply costs about $2—sometimes less if you get them from a clinic.

And most important, birth-control pills prevent the possibility of an accidental pregnancy. They're almost 100 percent effective when taken properly.

Many doctors, however, are reluctant to prescribe pills for young women unless they've been menstruating regularly for a year or two. A woman's body needs to develop its own natural hormone balance before that balance is interrupted by birth-control pills. So if you haven't been menstruating regularly for long, it's better to use another method of birth control for a while.

Although birth-control pills don't involve much work, they do involve certain responsibilities.

To start with, it's your responsibility to get complete information about taking the pills from the doctor. Many doctors skip the details when they discuss the pill because they assume young women won't understand them. But it's your body, so don't let an irresponsible doctor deny you the information you're entitled to. And when you see a doctor, it's a good idea to ask for the free instruction booklet written by the pill manufacturer.

You also have to be responsible about taking the pills. Birth-control pills should be taken at approximately the same time each day. Since it's easy to forget, it's a good idea to set up a schedule like taking the pill as soon as you get up or just before going to bed.

If you forget one pill, it must be taken as soon as you remember, even if this means taking two pills in the same day. One late pill usually will not interfere with your birth-control protection.

If you forget two pills in a row, take them both immediately, but use another method of birth control, like foam or condoms, until you get your next period.

It's possible to skip a period when you're taking birth-control pills. This is not necessarily a sign of pregnancy, so you should continue taking the next pack of pills on schedule. However, if you miss two periods in a row, you should see a doctor right away.

You should also return to the doctor or clinic for a checkup at least once a year. The doctor may not mention this, but it's very important, especially for young women. And you should report any unusual side effects when you go for a checkup.

Birth-control pills aren't perfect. They can't be used by every woman, and their side effects can be a problem. But for women who can use them safely and comfortably, the pills virtually eliminate the worry about an accidental pregnancy.

MORNING-AFTER PILLS

If a woman's egg has been fertilized by sperm, it travels down the fallopian tube and implants itself in the lining of the uterus. That's how a pregnancy normally starts.

But doctors have discovered that large doses of the female hormone estrogen, if taken on the day or two after intercourse, can prevent the fertilized egg from sticking to the uterus. And this stops a pregnancy that may have already begun.

Large doses of estrogen taken for this purpose are called morning-after pills. They are not a substitute for regular birth control, and they should be used only for emergency situations when something goes wrong with your usual method of birth control.

And this is certainly not a method of preventing pregnancy that a woman can use very often. The massive doses of estrogen are a thousand times greater than the dose in the normal birth-control pills, and they may produce dangerous side effects. In fact, there are many women who cannot take these pills at all, including women with a history of migraine headaches, hepatitis, blood clots, or heart disease.

Morning-after pills are also hard to get. Many doctors may not be familiar with them, and other doctors may be reluctant to prescribe such powerful pills to women under eighteen.

But if you've had unprotected intercourse or you think your birth-control method didn't work, it may be worth trying to get this pill in order to avoid a pregnancy or an abortion. Remember, however, that you have only a day or two in which to find a doctor or a clinic.

If you run across a sympathetic doctor who isn't familiar with morning-after pills, tell him the dosage recommended by the Health Department of Yale University is 50 milligrams of diethylstilbesterol taken once a day for five consecutive days. He'll be able to write a prescription for this, and you can get it filled at any drugstore.

It's also recommended that the doctor prescribe some kind of antinausea medicine, since taking the pills will probably cause severe vomiting and nausea.

Morning-after pills are a last resort, to be used only when other methods have failed. They are not a substitute for regular birth control, in fact, they're a lot more hassle. But they are something to keep in mind in case of emergency or accident.

METHODS THAT DON'T WORK

A lot of young women get pregnant every year by relying on techniques of birth control that don't work. Usually these ineffective techniques are based on myths or common misunderstandings about reproduction.

For example, one popular method of avoiding pregnancy is withdrawal. The man pulls his penis out of the vagina at the first sign of orgasm and ejaculates outside the woman's body. Some people think this prevents sperm from getting into the vagina.

But the drops of lubricating fluid released from the penis during sexual excitement and the early stages of intercourse may also contain sperm. Not much, but enough to get a woman pregnant.

Withdrawal does not work as birth control—it only interferes with sexual pleasure. And if you rely on this technique, pregnancy is inevitable.

Many women think they can prevent pregnancy by douching, or washing out the vagina, right after intercourse. But douching doesn't work, because sperm can enter the cervix a few seconds after ejaculation. And once sperm pass the cervix, they cannot be reached by any douche.

It doesn't matter what you douche with, nothing will work. Don't believe the myth that douching with Coca-Cola is effective. It's not—in fact, it can be very dangerous.

Another way many women try to avoid pregnancy is by using the rhythm method. It's a complicated technique based on avoiding intercourse around the time when a woman is supposed to be ovulating.

But it's impossible for a woman to tell when her egg is being released. And young women can't rely on this technique at all because they ovulate irregularly. Even with the supervised help of a doctor, most women who use the rhythm method will wind up getting pregnant.

Sometimes a woman may assume that the variety of "feminine-hygiene" products on the market can be used for birth control. In fact, manufacturers of these products often imply this in their advertising. But it's not true—these products are simply deodorants.

No spray or douching solution or suppository that's designed to make you smell pretty will give any protection against pregnancy. They may kill bacteria, but they won't kill sperm.

There are many other misconceptions about avoiding pregnancy. You may have heard that a woman can't get pregnant if she doesn't have an orgasm, if she urinates after intercourse, or if she fucks standing up. Some people even think that pregnancy can't occur the first time a woman has intercourse or unless she's in love.

Unfortunately getting pregnant doesn't have anything to do

with the way you feel or the way you fuck. It's simply a biological process that can happen any time sperm enters a woman's vagina.

There is no "natural" method of birth control. To avoid getting pregnant, you've got to use a birth-control device.

CHOOSING A METHOD

Choosing a method of birth control depends on your individual needs and life-style. There's no one method yet developed that's perfect for everybody.

In choosing among the various birth-control methods, there are several important considerations you should keep in mind:

How often do you have intercourse? The more frequently you have sex, the greater your chance of an accidental pregnancy. In general, the pills and IUD are designed for people who have intercourse regularly and need continual protection. Foams and condoms are probably most suitable for people who have sex only occasionally. The diaphragm can be used by either.

How much self-control is needed? There's no sense choosing a method of birth control that you won't use. Condoms, foams, and diaphragms require some planning and willpower, because you've got to use them correctly each time you have intercourse. Pills and IUDs are less hassle, since you don't have to think about them every time you have sex.

How reliable is each method? If you're seriously trying to avoid an accidental pregnancy, this is the most important question. Birth-control pills are the most effective. An IUD is the next best method, but many young women cannot use one. The diaphragm is very reliable if it's used properly. Condoms and foams are less reliable, but when used together, they're as effective as a diaphragm.

What are the side effects? Unfortunately the most reliable methods also have the most side effects. And many women are worried about using the pill or the IUD because of possible dangers. Condoms, foams, and diaphragms have no side effects, but they're liable to be a little messy to use.

How available is each method? Condoms and foams are easiest to get, especially if you're in a hurry. You must go to a doctor for pills, an IUD, or a diaphragm. But there are plenty of youth-oriented clinics around where you can get whatever kind of birth control you want.

Choosing a method of birth control requires careful thought and consideration, since each method has its advantages and disadvantages. Scientists are working on new methods like a male birth-control pill, a once-a-month pill, and even a vaccine that will make women immune to sperm for years. But none of these is available now and won't be for a long time. So the problem is choosing a reliable method of birth control right now that you feel comfortable with and that you'll use every time you have intercourse.

WHERE TO GET BIRTH CONTROL

In some states any minor has the right to get birth control without parental consent. In other states the laws are designed to make it difficult for minors to get the contraception they need.

To get a diaphragm, an IUD, or birth-control pills you must go to a doctor or clinic. The chart accompanying this section will tell you the provisions your state makes for minors when it comes to getting birth control without parental permission. As you can see, the laws vary from state to state.

If you live in a state where any minor is entitled to birth control, you have no problem. If you live in a state where there are no provisions for minors or where the laws are restrictive, chances are you'll still be able to find a doctor or clinic to help you.

For example, in New York and California, only certain minors

CONTRACEPTION: STATE LAWS

State health laws stipulate which minors are legally entitled to obtain contraception on their own consent without parents' knowledge or authorization.

ALABAMA: minors 14 or older

ALASKA: state laws unclear; it depends on the doctor or clinic

ARIZONA: married and emancipated minors

ARKANSAS: no provisions for any minor

CALIFORNIA: minors 15 and emancipated, married minors, pregnant minors

COLORADO: any minor

CONNECTICUT: no provision for any minor

DELAWARE: state laws unclear; it depends on the doctor or clinic

DISTRICT OF COLUMBIA: any minor

FLORIDA: any minor at the doctor's discretion

GEORGIA: any minor

HAWAII: no provision for any minor

IDAHO: no provision for any minor

ILLINOIS: any minor at the doctor's discretion

INDIANA: married and emancipated minors

IOWA: no provision for any minor

KANSAS: state laws unclear; it depends on the doctor or clinic

KENTUCKY: any minor

LOUISIANA: no provision for any minor

MAINE: no provision for any minor

MARYLAND: any minor

MASSACHUSETTS: no provision for any minor

MICHIGAN: no provision for any minor

MINNESOTA: emancipated minors

MISSISSIPPI: any minor

MISSOURI: married minors and parents

MONTANA: married minors

NEBRASKA: no provision for any minor

NEVADA: emancipated minors, married minors

NEW HAMPSHIRE: state laws unclear; it depends on the doctor or clinic

NEW JERSEY: married minors, pregnant minors

NEW MEXICO: emancipated minors, married minors

NEW YORK: married minors and parents

NORTH CAROLINA: emancipated minors

NORTH DAKOTA: no provision for any minor

OHIO: no provision for any minor

OKLAHOMA: no provision for any minor

OREGON: any minor

PENNSYLVANIA: pregnant minors, married minors, high school graduates

RHODE ISLAND: no provision for any minor

SOUTH CAROLINA: minors 16 or older

SOUTH DAKOTA: no provision for any minor

TENNESSEE: any minor

UTAH: no provision for any minor

TEXAS: married minors

VERMONT: no provision for any minor

VIRGINIA: any minor

WASHINGTON: no provision for any minor

WEST VIRGINIA: no provision for any minor

WISCONSIN: no provision for any minor

WYOMING: no provision for any minor

have the right to get birth control from a doctor on their own. But in reality there are many private doctors and clinics in both states that routinely treat any minor without parental consent.

In addition, most states have special provisions for treating minors in an emergency, and many doctors consider contraception an emergency for sexually active young women.

When it comes to condoms and spermicidal foams, they are sold in all drugstores without prescription. However, in some states the law actually forbids the sale of these products to minors under eighteen. If you have any trouble, you should lie about your age or try several different stores.

While it's good to know the laws in your state, it's not a good idea to take them too seriously. Getting the kind of birth control you want is just a matter of finding the right doctor or clinic. In most cities there are a variety of services that will help people under eighteen regardless of the law.

Private doctors. General practitioners, gynecologists, and internists can all prescribe birth control. However, gynecologists are usually more knowledgeable in this area, and they're more likely to treat women under eighteen without parental consent.

The only problem with gynecologists is that they're expensive—usually $15 to $25 or more a visit, and extra for the birth-control device. Bring a lot of cash if you don't want a bill to be sent to your home.

A Planned Parenthood survey of private doctors revealed that young doctors, urban doctors, and Jewish and Protestant doctors were more liberal about giving birth control to minors than their older, rural, or Catholic colleagues. This information could serve as a good guideline if you're trying to find a friendly doctor.

All the doctors in your city, including gynecologists, will be listed in the yellow pages under "Physicians."

Planned Parenthood. There are hundreds of Planned Parenthood clinics across the country, and the majority of these clinics treat women under eighteen without parental consent. Planned Parenthood is inexpensive, since the fees are usually based on what each patient can afford to pay. You can discuss each birth-control method with a nurse, and you'll be examined by a Planned Parenthood doctor.

Planned Parenthood is a good, reliable service. Because it's so popular, it's widely used, and the clinics are sometimes crowded. It may take a couple of weeks to set up an appointment, so don't call them the day before you need birth control.

Public health department and hospitals. The public health department in many cities operates neighborhood family-planning clinics, and so do many hospitals. They're often free, and many treat minors without parental consent.

Public clinics tend to be rushed and impersonal. But some cities have public clinics designed especially for women under eighteen, and these are usually more friendly. You can call your local health department and your local hospitals and ask about their family-planning services.

Free clinics and women's health centers. Many of these clinics provide birth-control services, and they rarely worry about age or parental consent. They're friendly and inexpensive. You can find them listed in underground newspapers or in the yellow pages under "Clinics."

Hotlines and switchboards. Many hotlines are designed specifically to help with this kind of problem. They'll usually be able to refer you to a reliable birth-control service in your area.

In the last chapter of this book there is a list of Planned Parenthood centers across the country. Free clinics, women's health centers, public health facilities, and hotlines in selected cities are also listed.

11

ABORTION

If a woman gets pregnant by accident, she has only two alternatives—having a baby or getting an abortion.

This is a very personal decision that every woman has to make for herself. But in general, having a baby presents too many problems for most young women. One way or another, the natural course of your life will be changed.

First, you'll have to quit school during your pregnancy. You may be forced into a premature marriage, or you may have to face the prospect of raising a child by yourself. Even if you decide to give the child away for adoption, your life will be upset, at least for a while.

On the other hand, having an abortion allows you to continue your life normally, postponing the experience of childbirth for later, when it can be a deliberate decision instead of an accident. For most young women abortion is the best alternative.

Abortion is a medical procedure that removes the fetus from the uterus before it's capable of living outside the woman's body. It's a simple operation, and it doesn't affect a woman's ability to get pregnant again in the future.

There are several misconceptions about abortion that make women afraid of having this operation. For example, women have been told that abortions are dangerous. But medical abortions performed by competent doctors are actually safer than having a child.

Women have also been told that abortions are emotionally harmful. But millions of women have had abortions and resumed their normal lives immediately and easily. In fact, the major emotional reaction is usually relief at ending a pregnancy that was an accident to begin with.

Although abortions are simple and safe, they should never be thought of as a substitute for birth control. After all, abortions are serious medical procedures, and they involve many problems.

In the first place, abortions are often hard to get. A complicated legal situation has limited the availability of abortions, especially when it comes to women under eighteen. The laws are presently changing, and abortions are becoming more widely available, but they're still a hassle to arrange, and in most parts of the country minors usually need their parents' permission.

Abortions are also very expensive. They can cost several hundred dollars, depending on where you live. Raising this kind of money is obviously difficult for a young woman who doesn't want to tell her parents she's pregnant.

There's no reason why abortions have to involve so many problems, since the operation itself is very simple. In other countries, like Japan and Russia, abortions are widely available with little expense and no hassle.

Our society, on the other hand, likes to punish people for having sex—especially young people. So arranging an abortion may involve some problems. But with a little determination you can get an abortion if you want one.

SELF-ABORTIONS

There is no way a woman can give herself an abortion. Anything you've ever heard about do-it-yourself abortion is a dangerous myth.

Some people think a pill exists that will bring on your period if you're pregnant. Doctors can make you menstruate with a dose of hormones, but only if you're not pregnant to begin with. There is no drug that will bring on a late period in a pregnant woman.

Women have tried swallowing handfuls of birth-control pills, quinine pills, or anything else they could find in an attempt to get rid of an accidental pregnancy. But medicines like these will not abort you—they'll only do severe damage to your body. In fact, there is nothing a woman can swallow to cause an abortion.

Countless women have died trying to abort themselves by sticking something inside the uterus to dislodge the fetus. Knitting needles, coat hangers, or any similar object can perforate the uterus, causing infection, hemorrhage, and death. Trying to suck the fetus out with a vacuum cleaner hose can kill you almost immediately.

Douching with dangerous substances like alcohol, lye, or cleaning fluid will not abort you. However, they will severely burn the inside of your vagina, and these douches can also kill you.

Some women try to induce an abortion by drinking enormous quantities of liquor. This will get you very stoned, but it won't get you unpregnant. Neither will sitting in a hot tub or jumping up and down. And throwing yourself down a flight of stairs can break all your bones without doing the least bit of damage to the fetus.

There is absolutely nothing a woman can do to bring about an abortion herself. Anything she tries may hurt her badly or even kill her.

Next to trying to abort yourself, the worst thing you can do is contact an unlicensed abortionist. Because safe, legal abortions are often hard to get, many people with little or no medical training have set themselves up in the illegal abortion business. These people, often called butcher abortionists, charge high fees and perform extremely dangerous, and often fatal, operations.

An abortion must be performed by a doctor who has special training in this kind of medical procedure. The safe abortion methods currently being practiced are described in this chapter, and they are the only types of abortion you should have.

ABORTION METHODS

Abortions are divided into two categories—early abortions, which are performed up to the twelfth week of pregnancy, and late abortions which are performed after the twelfth week of pregnancy.

Early abortions are safer, cheaper, and easier than late abortions. They take only about fifteen minutes, and they can be performed in a doctor's office or an out-patient clinic.

Late abortions, on the other hand, require staying in the hospital for a couple of days. They're expensive and complicated, and most hospitals will not perform late abortions on minors without parental consent.

So a woman who wants to have an abortion has got to act quickly in order to qualify for the early methods. This means having a pregnancy test as soon as your period is two weeks late. If the test is positive, you must start making abortion arrangements immediately. Don't put it off, because every day you wait brings you closer to the twelve-week point. Abortions can take several weeks to arrange, so you can't afford to lose any time.

The best early-abortion method is called vacuum aspiration. This quick, simple operation is performed with a special machine that sucks the fetus out of the uterus. It should not be confused with the household vacuum cleaner.

Before this abortion, a local anesthetic is injected into the back of the vagina, numbing that area of the body without putting you to sleep. Most women feel only minor discomfort during the operation, similar to menstrual cramps.

The first part of a vacuum aspiration abortion consists of dilating, or widening, the cervical opening. Normally the opening in the cervix is no bigger than the hole in a pierced ear. But with the use of special instruments the doctor stretches it to about the width of your thumb.

A hollow tube attached to the vacuum machine is then inserted through the cervix into the uterus. When the machine is turned on, the doctor passes the tube over the uterine walls until the fetus is sucked out of the body.

The whole process takes less than fifteen minutes. Afterward some women have cramps and want to lie down. Other women feel perfectly fine, but most clinics will have you rest for a while anyway.

Dilation and curettage, D&C for short, is another early-abortion method. D&C is a standard medical procedure used for many things besides abortions, such as removing abnormal growths on the uterus.

A woman will be anesthetized before this operation. While a local anesthetic is all that's needed, some doctors prefer to use general anesthetic, which puts you to sleep. The cervical opening is then dilated, as it is for a vacuum aspiration abortion.

During a D&C, the doctor scrapes the fetus away from the uterine wall with a spoonlike surgical instrument called a curretage. This is done carefully, to avoid damaging the uterus. The fetus is then removed from the body, and the abortion is over.

This operation usually takes about fifteen minutes. A woman may feel menstruallike cramps during and after a D&C performed with local anesthetic, and most women want to rest for a while before leaving the doctor's office.

After the twelfth week of pregnancy neither of these abortion methods can be used safely.

And late abortions are usually not performed until a woman is sixteen weeks pregnant. So in general, abortions are not done at all between the twelfth and the sixteenth week of pregnancy.

The late-abortion methods used once a woman is sixteen weeks pregnant are much more complicated than the early-abortion techniques. They involve staying in the hospital for several days and are therefore very expensive.

Saline injection is the most common late-abortion method. Instead of quickly removing the fetus, the doctor injects a solution through the abdomen and into the uterus. This brings on contractions in the uterus that cause a woman to expel the fetus herself.

It may take anywhere from a few hours to a few days before the contractions begin, and they may go on for several hours until the fetus is finally expelled. These uterine contractions are similar to the contractions of childbirth, and they can hurt.

Saline abortions have a few drawbacks. The injection doesn't always work the first time and may have to be repeated. Saline abortions also involve a higher risk of medical complications than the early methods.

The second late-abortion method is called hysterotomy, and it's the only method that involves actual surgery. Because this kind of abortion is so complicated, it's largely being replaced by the saline technique.

A hysterotomy is similar to a cesarean section performed to deliver a baby that cannot be born through the vagina. A small incision is made in the abdomen and in the uterus, and the fetus is removed. Because this operation is major surgery, a hysterotomy patient must stay in the hospital for about a week.

Most young women will not need a hysterotomy. And if abortion arrangements are made as soon as you find out you're pregnant, the saline method can be avoided too.

There is one more abortion method currently being practiced that has received a lot of publicity. It's called menstrual extraction, and it's really still in the experimental stage.

Menstrual extraction is a mini-abortion performed before a woman can tell if she's actually pregnant. It's done when your period is about a week late—too soon for a pregnancy to show up on the standard pregnancy test. So a woman who has a menstrual extraction never knows whether she was pregnant or whether her period was late for some other reason.

During menstrual extraction the uterine lining, or period, is drawn out through a special tube inserted through the cervix. If the woman is pregnant, the fertilized egg will come out with the period.

This process is quick and simple, but it has a lot of significant problems. Most important is the fact that you have no way of knowing whether you're really pregnant when a menstrual extraction is performed.

This is a special drawback for teenage women, since a young woman's menstrual cycle is often irregular to begin with, and a late period can mean a lot of things besides pregnancy. Menstrual extraction is best suited for women who have fairly regular cycles.

In addition, menstrual extraction doesn't always work on a woman who is pregnant. And this abortion technique can be painful, because anesthetic is generally not used.

If there is a doctor or clinic in your area that performs menstrual extractions, your local women's health center or abortion-referral agency may know about it. If you've had unprotected intercourse one month and your period doesn't come on time, you may want to look into this technique.

However, never try to perform menstrual extraction yourself. There are feminist organizations that advocate this and even sell the equipment needed. But even with the right equipment and careful instructions, you can hurt yourself badly. With the wrong equipment you can kill yourself.

Menstrual extraction, like every other kind of abortion, must be performed by a competent doctor.

AFTER AN ABORTION

Most women recover from early abortions very quickly. If the abortion is performed with local anesthetic, you may feel completely recovered in a matter of hours. Abortions performed with general anesthetic may leave you feeling tired for a couple of days, but in any case, a little rest is all that's needed.

Late abortions take longer to recover from. Saline abortions put your body through a lot of work and leave you feeling weaker than the simple early methods. A woman who has a late abortion may need a couple of days in bed to recuperate.

Some women feel depressed after an abortion. It's important to realize that depression is frequently a result of the changing level of hormones that takes place in the body after an abortion. It's a natural, temporary effect that soon disappears.

After an abortion a woman experiences menstruallike bleeding for several days. This bleeding is a normal part of the abortion process, and it's nothing to worry about. However, you're most prone to infection right after an abortion, so it's best to use sanitary napkins, not tampons, to absorb this blood flow.

Douching, exercise, and intercourse should all be avoided for a couple of weeks after an abortion. It's important to ask the doctor how long you must postpone these activities. The doctor may suggest you wait a week or two or until after your next period.

A woman will generally get her first period four to six weeks after an abortion. If it doesn't come for more than six weeks, it's a good idea to return to the doctor. A woman must also see the doctor if she develops a fever or very bad cramps in the days following the abortion, or if the postabortion bleeding is very heavy for more than ten days. These may be signs that something is wrong.

In most cases, though, nothing will go wrong. But it's a good idea to see a doctor anyway for a routine checkup after your first period. And this is also a good opportunity to find out about birth control.

It's important to realize that as soon as you've had an abortion, you're fertile, or capable of getting pregnant again. So you'll have to start making birth-control plans right away to avoid another accidental pregnancy.

Aside from being more careful about contraception, an abortion doesn't have to change your sex life at all. Abortions aren't fun, but they don't have to make you uptight about sex in general.

And nobody will be able to tell that you've had an abortion—not even a doctor can tell after the first few weeks. There's nothing different about your body that anyone can see or feel.

LEGAL STATUS OF ABORTION

If you're under eighteen, you may run into a variety of difficulties trying to arrange an abortion. And knowing a little about the legal status of abortion can help you deal with the difficulties.

Until recently abortions were illegal in most states except in special cases, and doctors could be arrested for performing them. But in January, 1973, the abortion situation changed.

The Supreme Court ruled that all women have the legal right to get abortions and that state governments could no longer prohibit them.

This ruling meant that the existing state laws against abortions were unconstitutional and would have to be changed. It also meant that doctors everywhere had the legal right to perform abortions, no matter what the state laws said.

So technically, abortions are totally legal throughout the country. But state governments have been very slow about changing their unconstitutional laws. In fact, many state legislators are determined to ignore the Supreme Court ruling and are trying to deny women their legal right to abortion. Of course, they can't get away with this forever, but it will take some time before every state can be forced to change.

In the meantime, abortions are becoming more and more available. Special abortion clinics are opening up in many cities, and private doctors are beginning to perform early abortions in their offices. But there are also many doctors and hospitals that are reluctant to do abortions even though they're legal, and abortions are still difficult to get in many parts of the country.

As usual, the situation is more complicated when it comes to women under eighteen. The Supreme Court didn't make any age requirements for abortions, but most states have general health laws that restrict all medical treatment for minors without parental consent.

A woman under eighteen has a much easier time getting an abortion if she has her parents' permission. With parental consent you're treated the same way as any woman over twenty-one. But without your parents' consent arranging an abortion is difficult in most states.

The majority of states require an unmarried woman to be eighteen to get an abortion on her own, and some states even insist you be twenty-one. Many states will allow a minor to get an abortion if she's emancipated, but that can be a hassle to prove.

Another problem for young women is the high cost of abortions. An early abortion costs about $125 in cities like New York and Los Angeles, where abortions are widely available, and as much as $350 in other parts of the country where abortion practice is limited. Late abortions are even more expensive and harder to get without parental consent.

WHERE TO GET AN ABORTION

The problems involved in arranging an abortion without telling your parents depend almost entirely on where you live.

Women who live in California will have the easiest time, because that state has granted all minors the legal right to obtain an abortion without parental permission. Abortions are widely available and relatively inexpensive—the average cost of an early abortion is $125.

To arrange an abortion in California the best place to call is your local Planned Parenthood. The telephone numbers for California Planned Parenthood centers are listed in the last chapter of this book.

In New York State abortions are completely legal, but most hospitals and clinics insist that a woman under eighteen have her parents' permission. Getting an abortion without parental consent is easier in New York City than in the rest of the state. Public hospitals in New York City will give an abortion to any woman who is seventeen or emancipated, and they'll sometimes give an abortion to a younger woman who can prove that telling her parents will "endanger her welfare."

In addition, there are a couple of private abortion clinics in New York City that have no requirements about age or parental consent. Planned Parenthood runs one of these clinics, and the Clergy Consultation Service will be able to refer you to other reliable clinics. The phone numbers for both of these organizations are listed in the last chapter of this book.

In most other cities getting an abortion is more difficult. Some cities, like Cleveland, don't have private abortion clinics, and the hospitals make it difficult for any woman, regardless of age, to arrange an abortion. In this case, your only alternative may be to travel to another city, and that's usually difficult to do without making your parents suspicious.

In many cities, like Washington, D.C., abortion is widely available, but the clinics are strict about requiring parental consent for women under eighteen. Sometimes it's possible to find a friendly doctor who will ignore the age restrictions. But if you can't, the only thing you can do is try lying about your age. If you look old enough, you may not be asked for proof.

If you can't pass for eighteen or emancipated, and you can't get away with traveling to another city, you'll probably have to get parental consent for an abortion.

However, if you don't want your parents to know about your sex life, you don't have to panic and tell them right away. It's best to first check out the available abortion facilities on your own, and there are two good national agencies that will help you do this:

Clergy Consultation Service on Abortion. Don't worry about the religious-sounding name. This nonprofit organization is the best abortion-referral service in the country. It's staffed by sympathetic counselors who are used to helping young people. Although many of the counselors are ministers, they're liberal and friendly, and they will never criticize your sex life or tell your parents.

The Clergy Consultation Service will have up-to-date information on the abortion facilities in your state. They'll be able to tell you if and where abortions are available without parental consent and how much they cost. You can be sure that the abortion facility they locate will offer the best, most inexpensive medical care in your area.

The counselor you speak to will be able to answer your questions about abortion and help with any problems you may have. If this agency can't find a clinic that doesn't require parental consent and you decide to tell your parents, the counselor will be happy to talk to your parents and help them accept your pregnancy and abortion.

The Clergy Consultation Service doesn't charge anything for their help, and they'll even try to get the abortion price lowered if you don't have any money.

There are Clergy Consultation Service chapters in twenty-nine states, and the phone number for each state is listed in the last chapter of this book. When you call these phone numbers, you may hear a recording telling you the name and number of the counselor nearest you. Since the Clergy Consultation Service is expanding, some of the phone numbers listed in this book may change by the time you need to use them. In that case, call the national office in New York for the latest number in your state. To reach the national office call: (212) 477-0034.

If the listings in this book don't include a Clergy Consultation Service chapter in your state, you can call the New York number below, and a Clergy Consultation Service worker will give you the name and phone number of an individual counselor in your area. For states not listed call: (212) 254-6314.

Planned Parenthood. Planned Parenthood has at least one office in almost every state, and most of these offices act as abortion-referral services. Some Planned Parenthood chapters even have their own abortion clinics.

Like the Clergy Consultation Service, Planned Parenthood is reliable and sympathetic. They will know if it's possible for you to get an abortion without parental consent, and the facility they recommend will provide good-quality medical care as inexpensively as possible.

Planned Parenthood also offers counseling to help with any problems you may have. If you don't have enough money for the abortion facility they find, Planned Parenthood will try to get the price lowered. And in places like New York and Los Angeles, where they run their own abortion clinics, the fees will be based on a sliding scale according to what you can afford.

Planned Parenthood offices across the country are listed in the last chapter of this book. There is also a national abortion-referral number run by Planned Parenthood that will help women from all over the country find safe abortions. If your local Planned Parenthood office can't help you, call: Family Planning Information Service at (212) 677-3040.

It's also possible to arrange an abortion by going directly to the facilities that perform them. You can call the following services in your area and ask about their fees and their policy toward minors:

Nonprofit abortion clinics. These special abortion clinics are opening up in many cities, and they will become more common as state laws change. They're generally reliable and relatively inexpensive, but they usually perform early abortions only. Nonprofit clinics sometimes advertise in newspapers, or you can find out about them from your local Clergy Consultation Service, Planned Parenthood, or the local women's health centers or hotlines in your areas.

Hospitals. Hospitals can always perform abortions, but they're generally conservative and tend to be strict about parental consent. Public hospitals have one advantage—they're usually not supposed to turn away patients who don't have any money. But at the same time the quality of health care in public hospitals is often inferior, and they put you through a lot of red tape.

Women's health centers and free clinics. Women's health centers sometimes perform abortions or work with a special abortion clinic. In general, the health care at women's centers is very good and as inexpensive as possible. Free clinics usually don't perform abortions, but they will probably be able to refer you to a good abortion clinic.

In trying to arrange the best abortion possible, there are also several places that a woman should avoid. Unfortunately these places are usually the ones that do a lot of advertising, so be careful about them:

Profit-making referral services. These agencies are opening up all over the country, charging high fees to refer you to an abortion clinic. Often the clinics they recommend are unnecessarily expensive. In fact, profit-making referral services have been made illegal in New York because of their rip-off tactics. There's no reason to call these places, since there are nonprofit services available.

Profit-making abortion clinics. While these clinics may be perfectly competent, they often charge very high fees. Some profit-making clinics have been known to tell a woman she's pregnant when she really isn't, in order to charge her for an unnecessary abortion.

If you're calling up clinics advertised in local newspapers, don't hesitate to ask if they're profit-making or nonprofit. If you go to a profit-making clinic, it's a good idea to have a pregnancy test done elsewhere first, so you know you aren't being ripped off.

Birthright. Birthright is a Catholic organization with branches in many cities, and they do a lot of advertising. Sometimes their ads make them sound like an abortion-referral service, but they are not.

Birthright is opposed to abortion, and they'll do anything they can to prevent you from having one. They'll try to make you feel guilty and frightened about having an abortion in order to convince you to carry out your pregnancy.

If a woman doesn't want to have an abortion, Birthright can be helpful about arranging for unwed mother's homes and adoption facilities. But if you do want an abortion or if you haven't made up your mind, do not go to this organization. They'll try to make up your mind for you.

Check the last chapter of this book for the Planned Parenthood office and the Clergy Consultation Service chapter nearest you. Women's health centers, free clinics, and hotlines in your area may also be able to refer you to a reliable abortion clinic.

12

CARE AND FEEDING OF SEX ORGANS

Your sex organs aren't very different from the rest of your body. In addition to some pleasant exercise, they need to be kept reasonably clean, and occasionally they need medical attention.

Many of us, however, are brought up to regard our sex organs as a totally separate part of our anatomy—something that shouldn't be touched or talked about like the rest of our body. And this can cause all kinds of problems.

While we're bombarded with information on cleaning our teeth and clearing our complexions, very little is ever said about how to take care of our genitals. So some people are careless, other people are overly cautious, and everybody is a little embarrassed.

And when something goes wrong with our sex organs, it's

usually twice as frightening as any other kind of illness because we don't know what it is or what to do about it.

Nobody is told very much about their genitals. And most people have to learn to take care of themselves as they go along. But it's easier if you know what kind of problems to expect and what to do about them.

SOAP AND WATER

The sex organs need to be washed regularly to keep them clean and healthy. You don't have to be a cleanliness freak, but you do have to use a little soap and water.

For one thing, the skin of the genitals, like the skin on the rest of the body, tends to sweat. But unlike the rest of the body, the genitals are usually covered all day with several layers of clothing. This means air can't circulate, and the genitals tend to stay damp—which makes an ideal breeding ground for bacteria.

And bacteria are what cause everything from infections to odors. The genitals usually have a slight smell, but when they're clean, the smell is fresh and pleasant, like clean hair. It's only when the sex organs get sweaty and musty from not being washed that the odor can get unpleasant.

The genitals also secrete natural oils to keep the delicate skin soft and lubricated. But these oils can collect into a sticky white substance if you don't bathe regularly. Men who aren't circumcised should always pull back the foreskin of the penis when washing because oils tend to collect there. And women should clean in the folds of the vaginal lips and around the clitoris for the same reason.

Aside from soap and water, nothing else is needed for a man or woman to keep clean. A great deal has been made out of "feminine hygiene"—mostly for the purpose of selling women unnecessary products. Advertisements usually imply that a woman's genitals are some kind of special problem to keep clean, but that's total nonsense.

The inside of the vagina tends to clean itself naturally. Menstrual flow, lubricating fluids, even semen all drain out of the vagina. A woman needs only to wash the outside of the vagina, and the inside will take care of itself.

Many women have been told that it's necessary to douche regularly. Douching is simply rinsing out the inside of the vagina. This is usually done with the aid of a rubber douche bag or douching syringe.

Sometimes douching is part of a treatment prescribed by a doctor to cure a minor vaginal infection, but that's the only time it's medically necessary. As far as birth control goes, douching is absolutely useless.

However, a woman might want to douche her vagina after menstruation or after intercourse. Occasional douching is all right, but douching too often can be harmful.

The inside of a healthy vagina contains natural bacteria and acids that kill germs and ward off infections. Douching too much washes away these acids and makes a woman more susceptible to a variety of infections.

If a woman wants to douche once in a while, she should avoid using any of the commercial douching powders and liquids sold in drugstores. Many of them contain harsh chemicals that can only irritate the delicate vaginal skin. A quart of plain water with a tablespoon of clear vinegar is the best douching solution a woman can use. The vinegar helps restore the natural acids that water washes away.

In fact, it's a good idea for a woman to avoid all the drugstore products for "feminine hygiene." At best these products are rip-offs, and some of them are downright harmful.

One product that's being hyped a lot is vaginal deodorant spray. These sprays are totally unnecessary and can irritate the vaginal lips. They should never be used. If you want to smell especially good, a drop of perfume in the pubic hair is much better.

But all a woman—or a man—really needs for healthy, clean-smelling genitals is regular washing. Manufacturers and advertisers would like to convince you that your sex organs are "dirty" without their useless products. Save your money, your sex organs are beautiful all by themselves.

MENSTRUATION

Menstruation is a healthy and normal part of a woman's reproductive cycle. Like many other body processes, it can involve some minor discomfort and inconvenience. But since menstruation has to do with sex, the minor problems are often greatly exaggerated, and a multitude of myths have developed about menstruation.

Women have been told they can't bathe, be physically active, or have sex during their period. Ridiculous restrictions like these make people think of menstruation as an illness. In reality, bathing, exercise, and sex are as necessary and healthy during menstruation as they are during the rest of the month. There's nothing a woman cannot do just because she has her period.

Some people think a menstruating woman is weak because she's losing blood. But there are only two or three ounces of blood in an average period, and that's not enough to even notice. Besides, the body naturally replaces that blood very quickly.

Of course there is some real inconvenience associated with menstruation. When a woman first starts menstruating, her periods are usually very unpredictable, and that can cause a lot of anxiety. Every woman's menstrual cycle is unique, and it may take months or even years before a woman establishes her own pattern.

In addition, there are a variety of physical effects that may accompany a woman's period. Most of these are a result of the changing balance of hormones in the body, and they're perfectly normal.

Constipation or diarrhea, backaches, headaches, and pimples are some of the things that can occur on the days before or during menstruation. They may be a nuisance, but they're rarely a serious problem.

A woman may notice a slight weight gain right before her period, and her breasts may swell and become sensitive. This happens because the body retains fluids during menstruation. The bloated feeling you get from fluid retention can be mildly uncomfortable, but it's certainly not harmful.

Menstrual cramps are probably the biggest problem for many women. They're very common, but in most cases cramps aren't severe and they don't interfere with a woman's normal activities.

While cramps can be a real physical discomfort, they can also have something to do with a woman's attitude toward her period. If a woman is expecting pain, her muscles become tense, and she'll probably feel worse cramps than a woman who is relaxed. That's why exercise is often recommended to reduce cramps. And sex can do the same thing, since orgasms are a good form of muscle-relaxing exercise.

Not all women experience discomfort during menstruation, but many women do. There's no reason for a woman to think she's sick during her period. In fact, getting a period is a healthy sign that the body is working properly. And sexually active women are usually happy when they menstruate, because it means they're not pregnant.

However, advertisers of the many useless menstrual products like to exaggerate the discomforts and play up the myths about menstruation. Magazines and television are constantly promoting pills that supposedly relieve cramps, vitamins that claim to replace iron lost through menstruation, and a host of deodorizing products that capitalize on the fear of odor.

If a woman sees enough of these ads, she's bound to get the impression that menstruation is a terrible, embarrassing problem. And that's what the advertisers are counting on.

But all of these products are bullshit. If a woman wants to reduce cramps, she needs only a couple of aspirin. If the cramps are really severe, she should see a doctor. Any woman who has an iron deficiency should also see a doctor, and not rely on the claims of a commercial vitamin.

Advertisers are most deceptive when it comes to the myth about menstrual odor. When menstrual blood comes in contact with air, it produces a slight smell, but not enough for anyone to notice. Nobody can tell if a woman has her period. If sanitary napkins are changed a few times a day, the odor doesn't have a chance to build up, and if tampons are used, the possibility of odor is eliminated.

Tampons are more convenient than napkins for a lot of reasons. They fit snugly into the vagina, where they can't be seen or felt, and tampons absorb the menstrual flow much better than napkins do. Tampons are easy to insert, they're perfectly safe, and a woman can use them even if she's a virgin because there are natural holes in the hymen that can usually admit a tampon.

Changing tampons and bathing regularly are all that's needed to keep clean and healthy during menstruation. A period doesn't involve any extra hygiene or special restrictions, and a woman can be as active and free during menstruation as she is the rest of the month.

COMMON AILMENTS AND INFECTIONS

The sex organs, like any other part of the body, are subject to a number of common ailments and infections that require medical attention.

Many people, however, are embarrassed about going to a doctor when anything is wrong with their genitals. They assume that any ailment must come from fucking. But that's not true. There are several common infections you can get whether you're having sex or not.

In general, women seem to be more susceptible to genital infections than men. Because the vagina is an opening in the body, it is easy for germs to enter. And its moist, warm climate makes a perfect place for bacteria to grow.

The first sign of a vaginal infection is usually an abnormal discharge from the vagina. The healthy vagina produces a small amount of clear or milky odorless liquid. If a woman suddenly develops a very heavy discharge, one that itches, smells, or is a different color, she probably has some kind of infection.

One common form of vaginal infection, called monilia, comes from yeast. Yeast grows naturally in the healthy vagina, together with certain harmless kinds of bacteria and acids that keep the yeast under control. If anything upsets this natural balance, the yeast can start multiplying and cause a problem.

This infection does not come from having sex. A yeast infection can develop on its own anytime the climate in the vagina changes.

Wearing tight clothing and panty hose are often blamed for causing yeast infections because they keep the vagina excessively damp. Taking antibiotics to cure an illness somewhere else in the body is another common cause. The drugs kill off the healthy bacteria in the vagina that keep the yeast from spreading.

And taking birth-control pills also changes the normal climate in the vagina and encourages the growth of yeast. Women on the pill often have a continual problem with yeast infections.

Although monilia is not dangerous, it's very annoying. As yeast multiplies inside the vagina, it produces a thick, white discharge. This discharge can irritate the vaginal lips and is liable to cause severe itching.

The only way to get it cleared up is to see a doctor to have it properly diagnosed and treated. The usual treatment includes putting medicated tablets into the vagina every day for several weeks. That cures a mild case, but yeast infections are extremely common and often recur.

Another widespread vaginal infection is trichomonas—usually called "trich" for short. It's caused by a one-celled bug that's found very frequently in both men's and women's genitals.

In men, trichomonas is usually harmless and causes no symptoms. But in women the infection produces a foamy vaginal discharge, which is yellowish in color and very unpleasant smelling. As the discharge drains from the body, it irritates the vaginal lips and causes continual itching.

It's possible to pick up a trich infection from wet towels or dirty clothing, but it's also passed back and forth between men and women during intercourse. If a woman finds she has this infection, it's important that her sexual partner be treated too. Otherwise she will just get the infection again the next time they have sex together.

Trichomonas is cured by taking a prescription drug called Flagyl several times a day for about two weeks. Persistent infections may also require using medicated tablets inside the vagina.

There are a number of other common infections of the vagina that are usually lumped together under the name nonspecific vaginitis. That's what doctors call any infection that causes a discharge or an itch but can't be identified.

And since doctors don't know what it is, they can't tell what causes it. But most minor infections, regardless of what they may be, can be cleared up with antibiotics and vaginal medication.

Another common area of infection, in men as well as women, is the urinary system. Although the reproductive system and the urinary system have totally separate functions, they're located right next to each other, and in men they even share some of the same organs, like the penis.

An infection can occur anywhere along the urethra or in the bladder. Urinary infections cause a painful burning sensation when you piss, and you'll feel like you have to piss all the time. A discharge from the urethra is also a common symptom, especially in men.

Doctors don't know what causes most cases of urinary infection, so they call them nonspecific urethritis. That means there is some infection in the urethra, but they can't isolate the germ, nor can they explain how you got it.

Some urinary infections can come from having sex, but it's also possible to pick up urethritis when you're not having sex at all.

Most urinary infections are treated with antibiotics, although it may take several weeks to clear up a troublesome case. If you do have a urinary infection, you should make sure your sexual partner gets medical treatment too. If you don't, the infection will just keep moving back and forth between the two of you and it will flare up again.

Men can also get an inflammation in the prostate gland. It can come from a number of things, including an infection in the urinary system or a sudden change in the amount of sexual activity.

The symptom of a prostate inflammation are painful and unpleasant—a burning sensation when you piss, a discharge from the penis, and possibly a dull pain in the testicles or rectum.

One other pest that's fairly common for both men and women is crabs—a small crab-shaped form of lice that live in the pubic hair and drive you crazy with itching. You can get crabs from someone you sleep with, or you can get them from infested clothing or bedding.

If you come down with an unexplained itching in your pubic hair, look around for the tiny bugs. They're usually big enough to see with the naked eye.

Although crabs are extremely unpleasant and uncomfortable, they're easy to get rid of. All you have to do is coat the pubic area with a lice-killing cream or liquid. Three common brands that are available in any drugstore without a prescription and cost less than $2 are Cuprex, Barc, and Pyrinate A-200. If two applications of these lice killers don't do the job, then you should see a doctor to get a prescription for a stronger medicine.

Aside from crabs, all the common infections mentioned here are liable to produce symptoms very similar to those of venereal disease. VD can produce a discharge or a burning itch, just like a vaginal infection or an inflammation of the urethra.

But you can get venereal disease only from having sex. If you haven't had intercourse, then you don't have VD. If you have had intercourse, then you can't always tell what the problem is. The important thing is to go to a doctor or clinic whenever you have any unusual discharge, soreness, or itching in the genitals. Minor infections are very common, everybody gets them sometime or other. And the only way to get rid of infections is to have them properly diagnosed and treated.

But it's important to remember that doctors aren't always very clear in their explanations. So you should ask what exactly you have, how you got it, and whether or not you can have intercourse while you're being treated.

To cure an infection in the vagina, the urinary system, or the prostate, you usually have to refrain from intercourse while you're being treated. But doctors don't always tell you this, especially if you're young.

It's your body, however, so make sure you get complete instructions and then follow them carefully.

GYNECOLOGICAL EXAMINATION

Women need medical attention more often than men do when it comes to taking care of the sex organs. For one thing, women seem to get genital infections more frequently. And women also have to see doctors for pregnancy tests and menstrual problems —areas that don't affect men.

Annual medical examinations are necessary for women using a diaphragm, an IUD, or birth-control pills. And it's a good idea for every woman to have a yearly test for cancer of the cervix—a disease that can usually be cured if it's detected early enough.

The branch of medicine that deals specifically with the female reproductive system is called gynecology. When you have a gynecological examination, two parts of your body are checked —the breasts and the sex organs.

If you have this examination done at a clinic, you may be treated by a gynecologist, a general practitioner, or an internist. But if you go to a private doctor, it's best to choose a gynecologist. They generally know more about the various genital infections, and they're usually more liberal about sex and birth control.

Some women hesitate to get the kind of medical care they need simply because they're afraid of having their genitals examined. But a gynecological examination isn't painful, and it takes only a few minutes. It shouldn't be a frightening experience, especially if you know what to expect beforehand.

The first part of the examination consists of taking your medical history. You'll be asked about diseases you've had and diseases that run in your family. The doctor will want to know about your menstrual periods—how old you were when you started menstruating, how regular your periods are, and the date of your last period. You may also be asked a few questions about your sexual experience.

After the medical history is taken, you'll be asked to undress for the examination. The doctor will check your breasts by gently pressing and feeling them, to detect any abnormal lumps that may be a sign of cancer. The breast exam is usually done once as you sit on the examining table and again after you lie down.

The pelvic examination to check the sex organs is done as you lie with your feet in stirrups on the end of the examining table. Your legs are spread apart, so the entire area of your vulva is visible.

This is the awkward part of the examination. It's good to

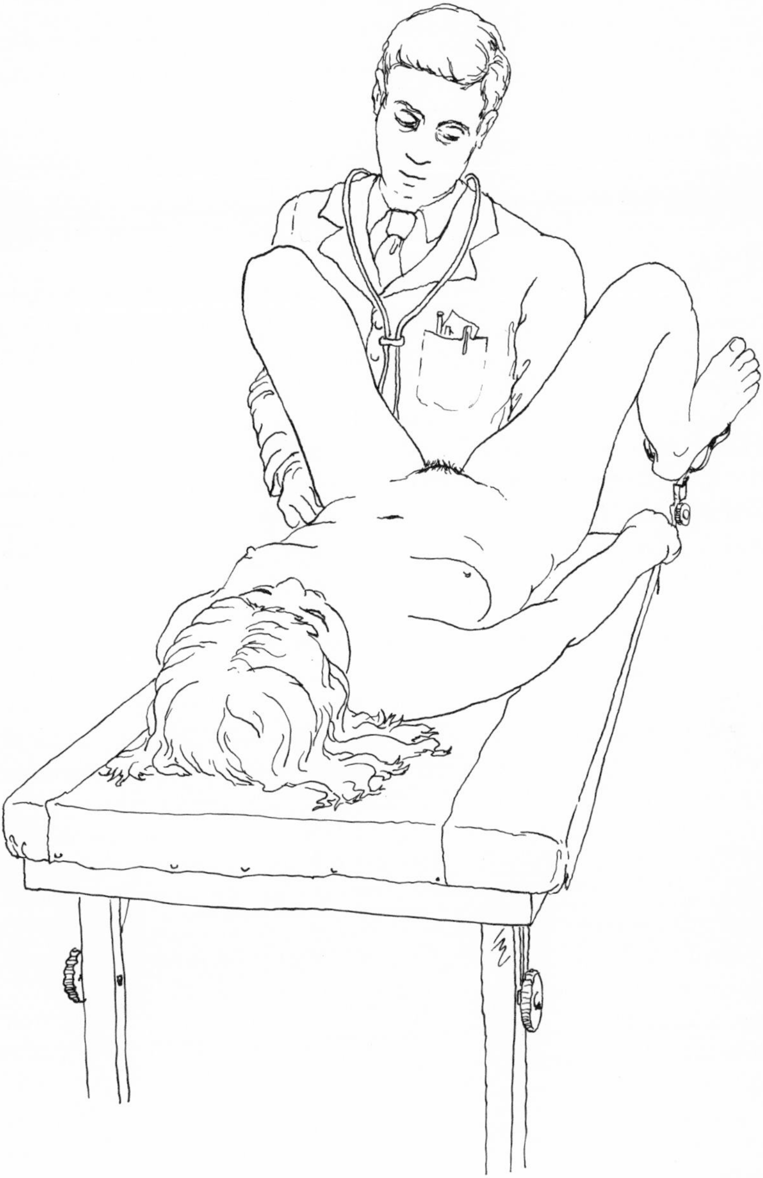

keep in mind that the doctor has done this thousands of times and realizes this examination can be embarrassing for a young woman. So try to relax.

The doctor will check your uterus and other internal organs by inserting a gloved finger into your vagina, while pressing the other hand against your abdomen. Sometimes the doctor will also check the position of these organs by inserting a finger into your anus, a procedure which may feel a little uncomfortable.

A speculum will then be inserted into your vagina. This a hollow metal or plastic tube that holds the vaginal walls apart, allowing the doctor to see your cervix and check for signs of irritation.

With the speculum still in place, you'll be given a Pap test for cervical cancer. A cotton swab is inserted into your cervical opening to collect some cells, and the cells are smeared on a glass slide that will be sent to a laboratory for analysis. Having a Pap smear taken is quick and painless.

A second smear should also be taken to test for gonorrhea. But most doctors will not do this automatically, so if you want a gonorrhea test, you'll have to ask for it.

Assuming everything is normal and healthy, your gynecological examination will be over at this point. The whole procedure usually takes ten to fifteen minutes, and most women leave the doctor's office feeling relieved and happy to know that their body is working properly. Returning for the next checkup is always easier.

It's important that each gynecological examination you have be as thorough as possible. And there are several ways you can make sure of this.

Never douche before the examination. Douching will only wash away any signs of infection that may be present in your vagina, and the examination will be pretty useless. The doctor will want to see how your vagina looks in its natural state.

And if you're having a checkup for a specific reason, like birth control or a VD test, explain that before you're examined. Doctors rarely ask specific questions, and they assume you want only a routine exam if you don't speak up.

It's also your responsibility to mention any unusual symptoms you have, like a discharge, an itch, or a burning sensation when you piss. Painful intercourse is sometimes a result of vaginal infections, so if having sex makes the entrance of your vagina hurt it's important to mention this too. The doctor needs your help to diagnose a problem.

And don't be afraid to ask questions about the examination and about your body. Doctors don't usually volunteer much information, but it's your right to know what each part of the exam is for and what the doctor finds out about you. If you're being treated for an infection, you'll want to know as much as possible.

Asking questions during a gynecological exam is a good way to learn about your genitals. Another way to learn about your body is self-examination, a concept that has developed in the women's movement. Many women are doing their own modified version of a pelvic exam by inserting a speculum into the vagina and looking at the cervix through a mirror.

It's interesting and educational to see the inside of your vagina and cervix, as long as you're careful not to hurt yourself with the speculum. But it's not possible to diagnose infections by yourself, and self-examination is certainly not a substitute for periodic visits to the doctor.

WHERE TO GET MEDICAL HELP

Sooner or later, everybody who's sexually active needs to see a doctor. But getting medical help when you need it can often be a hassle for minors.

To diagnose a genital infection properly or even to give a routine gynecological examination, a doctor should know whether or not you're having intercourse. And since it's not a good idea to lie about stuff like that, you may want to avoid the family doctor—especially if you think you've picked up an infection from fucking.

But getting medical care on your own presents other problems. There are all kinds of complicated and contradictory state laws about giving minors any kind of medical treatment without their parents' permission.

Fortunately there are lots of loopholes in these laws that allow doctors to treat a minor in an emergency or when the attempt to get parental consent might endanger the minor's health. A sympathetic doctor can always use these loopholes to help you.

In addition, most cities have clinics that treat minors on their own consent. And you can usually get routine sexual health care without involving your parents if you just know where to look.

Private doctors. Urologists are specialists who treat urinary infections, but men can usually go to any general practitioner, and women can get most of their health-care needs taken care of by a gynecologist. All of these doctors are listed in your local phone book under "Physicians."

Private doctors are expensive. Costs can run anywhere from $10 to $40 a visit, and extra if laboratory fees are necessary to diagnose an infection. You'll have to pay the doctor right away in cash if you don't want a bill sent to your home. And you'll need more money to pay for any medication the doctor prescribes.

The high cost of private doctors makes this an impossible alternative for many people in our society, not just for minors.

Free clinics. There are free clinics in many cities across the country that give medical help to young people and others who can't afford private doctors. They're usually staffed by dedicated young doctors, and there's no hassle about age or parental consent.

Free clinics can often be found by checking your local underground newspaper or the yellow pages under "Clinics."

Women's health centers. Women's health centers and clinics have formed in many cities with the specific purpose of giving women good gynecological health care at minimal cost. These groups will usually treat you on your own consent, regardless of state laws.

You can find women's health centers in your area by checking local underground newspapers or the yellow pages or by contacting a local women's liberation organization.

Public health clinics. In most cities the public health department operates clinics that are free or very cheap. Hospitals often have public clinics, too.

Public clinics are often crowded and impersonal, and they may not provide the best medical service available. It's a good idea to call any public clinic in advance, explain what you want, and ask if they treat people your age without parental consent.

Planned Parenthood. The main purpose of Planned Parenthood is to provide birth control. When a woman goes to Planned Parenthood for a birth-control device, she'll get a breast examination, a pelvic examination, and a Pap test. But a woman cannot get these services unless she's already a birth-control patient, and Planned Parenthood will usually not treat any kind of genital infections.

However, your local Planned Parenthood might be able to recommend a good clinic or doctor for general medical care.

Hotlines. Youth-oriented hotlines in your area will be able to recommend a doctor or clinic that will give you the medical care you're looking for.

Hotlines, free clinics, women's health centers, public clinics, and Planned Parenthoods in many cities are listed in the last chapter of this book.

13

VENEREAL DISEASE

Venereal disease is the number one health problem of our generation. It infects more people than any other illness besides the common cold. Each year close to 3 million people get VD—and the majority of them are under the age of twenty-five.

The two most common kinds of venereal disease are syphilis and gonorrhea. They're both highly contagious, and they're spread from person to person by having sex.

VD is not a moral disease. It's not caused by "promiscuity" or poverty or prostitutes. Syphilis and gonorrhea are simply contagious diseases—no more serious and no less serious than a dozen other diseases you could catch.

The only unique feature of venereal disease is how it spreads. Both syphilis and gonorrhea are caused by germs that need constant warmth and moisture in order to survive. And the only warm moist parts of the human body that provide a suitable environment for these germs are the sex organs, the mouth, and the anus.

In order for VD to get from one person to another, you need direct physical contact between these parts of the body. That means VD can be spread only during intercourse, anal intercourse, or oral sex. While it's possible in some special cases to transmit VD from mouth to mouth kissing it's highly unusual.

Syphilis and gonorrhea germs cannot live outside the human body for more than a few seconds. This makes it impossible to catch VD from a toilet seat, a dirty towel, or a drinking glass. The germs die too quickly on contact with air. You can get VD only from a person who has it—and only then if your warm, moist parts come in contact with their warm, moist parts. Shaking hands with somebody is not enough, no matter how hot and sweaty your hands may be.

Syphilis and gonorrhea aren't the only illnesses you can catch from sex. You can get a cold or measles or mononucleosis or lots of other things from sleeping with somebody who has them. But most diseases are transmitted through the air or through contaminated objects. VD is different—the germs go directly from one person's genitals to the other's during intercourse.

And while it may be fun catching VD, it's no fun having it. Both syphilis and gonorrhea can cause painful, unpleasant symptoms. If left untreated, they can do permanent damage to your body.

What makes venereal disease even more dangerous is that many people don't know they have it. Women especially may not notice any signs of VD until it has created serious complications.

It's easy for a woman to catch VD and pass it on to her sex partner without even suspecting that she's infected. And if her partner has intercourse with several other people, each of them can catch it. Before you know it, hundreds of people are walking around with VD. This is how the diseases spread.

Despite the invention of antibiotics, which can stop VD quickly and cheaply, there has been a tremendous increase in the amount of VD during the last ten years. Most of this increase has been due to the spread of gonorrhea. In fact, so many people have gonorrhea today that health authorities call it an epidemic.

And young people are the major victims of this epidemic.

Nationwide it's estimated that one out of every fifty high school students has gonorrhea. In cities like San Francisco, Atlanta, and Washington, D.C., it's more like one out of every twenty. And health officials say that if the present rate continues in California, one out of every two high school students will have gonorrhea by 1980.

There are lots of reasons for this epidemic. For one thing, widespread use of the birth-control pill has probably helped spread gonorrhea. Previously most people relied on condoms for birth control, and condoms also provide protection against catching and transmitting VD.

The pill also changes the climate inside a woman's vagina. Normally there are certain acids inside the vagina that help kill off germs, but the pill eliminates these acids and helps create a more hospitable climate for gonorrhea infection.

The war in Vietnam has also played a part. Soldiers returning from Vietnam have brought home new strains of gonorrhea that are more resistant to antibiotics. Routine treatment with penicillin has been killing off the weaker kinds of gonorrhea, but the stronger types survive and continue to spread.

But the major reason for the spread of VD is fear and ignorance. Most people are taught nothing about venereal disease at home and very little in school. Young people simply do not get the information they need to protect themselves—because supposedly "responsible adults" are too embarrassed to talk about sex.

You can be sure that if we had an epidemic of flu or smallpox or polio, something would be done about it. But because VD is connected with sex, the whole subject is ignored.

Young people also have more VD because they have less access to good medical care. Not only are doctors expensive, but most states have legal restrictions against minors getting routine medical care on their own. So young people see doctors less often and walk around with more gonorrhea.

And finally, doctors themselves are not doing the job they should. Despite the current epidemic of gonorrhea, doctors will rarely suggest a VD exam. So people walk into their office with a sore throat and gonorrhea and walk out with the gonorrhea unnoticed.

The only advice that most parents and schools offer about VD is "Don't fuck." That may be one way of avoiding infection, but it makes the remedy sound worse than the disease.

It makes more sense to assume that if you're sexually active you're going to get a dose of VD sooner or later. And the best thing to do is know something about these diseases—how to reduce your risks, how to recognize the symptoms, and where to get medical help quickly.

The principal danger is not in catching venereal disease—the danger lies in ignoring it.

SYPHILIS

Syphilis is an ancient disease that's been around in one form or another ever since man evolved from the ape. And from time to time throughout history, epidemics of the disease have crippled and killed millions of people.

Despite the fact that modern antibiotics are able to stop syphilis, it's still a serious health problem. About 100,000 cases of syphilis are reported every year—which is much smaller than the number of gonorrhea cases. But health officials estimate that there may be half a million people walking around with syphilis who don't know it.

Syphilis infection usually starts in the genitals, but the disease can attack every organ in your body. If treated early, it can be easily cured, but if it's not treated, the disease will do serious and permanent damage. What makes syphilis even more dangerous is the fact that you can have the disease for months or even years without noticing any symptoms.

Syphilis is caused by a tiny spiral-shaped germ that thrives on the moist tissues of the sex organs, the anus, and the mouth. It can be transmitted by any direct contact between these three areas of the body, but usually it's spread by intercourse.

The syphilis germ moves like a twisting corkscrew, and during intercourse with an infected person, the germ bores right through the skin of the new victim's sexual organs. Within hours, the infection has established a new home and begun to multiply.

If syphilis goes unnoticed or untreated, the disease will progress through three distinct stages.

The first sign of syphilis infection, which occurs anywhere from ten days to three months after intercourse with an infected person, is the appearance of a chancre.

The chancre (pronounced shanker) is a hard red bump on the skin. It may look like a pimple, a blister, or a cold sore, but usually it's painless.

The chancre appears on that part of the body where the syphilis germs broke through the skin. On men this is usually on the head of the penis, although it can be anywhere on the shaft of the penis or the scrotum.

In women the chancre usually develops on the cervix or along the walls of the vagina. And since this little red bump usually doesn't hurt, it's extremely difficult for a woman to tell if she's infected.

If syphilis germs are transmitted during anal intercourse, the chancre will grow somewhere inside the rectum. Again, it's difficult or impossible to notice.

And if you get syphilis by kissing or sucking the genitals of an infected person, the chancre may appear on your lips, your tongue, or your tonsils.

During this first stage syphilis is highly contagious. The chancre is filled with millions of teeming syphilis germs. Any discharge or pus from the chancre is highly infectious, so it should never be squeezed or scratched, since you could spread the germs around.

If you don't get treated, the syphilis chancre will disappear by itself in a few weeks. You may think the problem is cleared up, but in fact the disease is just progressing to the second stage. Syphilis germs, carried by the bloodstream, now spread throughout the body.

A few weeks after the chancre disappears, a measleslike skin rash develops. This rash can appear anywhere: on the chest, shoulders, back, arms, legs, on the genitals, or even on the palms of your hands or the soles of your feet. Regardless of where the rash appears or how long it lasts, it usually doesn't itch or hurt.

In addition to the rash, some people also develop a sore throat, swollen glands, a low fever, or headaches. You may feel generally sick and nauseous as though you had the flu.

This stage of the disease can last anywhere from two weeks to two months, and during this time the infection is highly contagious.

But it's important to remember that almost half of all women who have syphilis don't show either the primary or the secondary symptoms. In other words, there's no chancre, no rash, no feeling of being sick. Nevertheless, they have the disease and can pass it on to anybody they have sex with.

If syphilis isn't cured at this stage, all the external symptoms will go away by themselves. For the next ten or twenty years a person may not even suspect that anything is wrong.

But inside the body, syphilis continues to attack the vital organs. It can spread to the liver, the lungs, the eyes, the heart, or the brain. And years after the original infection, sometimes as long as twenty or thirty years, syphilis can suddenly manifest itself in organ damage, heart attack, blindness, insanity, or even death.

But it's very unusual for anyone in this country to let syphilis develop to the final stage. Even if there are no symptoms to send people running to a doctor, syphilis often gets discovered during routine blood tests such as those required for a marriage license or blood donation. And many people get cured of syphilis without even knowing they had it when they take massive doses of antibiotics to cure some other illness.

Syphilis can be discovered and stopped anywhere along the line. But if the disease has had years to destroy your internal organs, the damage cannot be repaired.

Recognizing syphilis, however, isn't always easy. The symptoms—if there are any—can resemble a dozen other things. You might have a little rash for a few days or a fever, but then everything seems to clear up. You stop worrying, but the trouble has just begun.

So if you have any reason to suspect you may have syphilis—any hard red pimple on your genitals, any unexplained rash that doesn't itch—go to a doctor or clinic immediately. If you delay until the symptoms disappear, it will only make the disease more difficult to diagnose.

There are two standard ways of diagnosing syphilis. First, if you happen to have any chancre or open sore, a doctor can take some of the fluid out and examine it under a microscope to find the syphilis germs.

The second and most common method is a blood test. A small amount of blood is taken from your arm and sent to a lab for analysis. It's important to remember, however, that this test is not completely reliable unless you've had the disease for four or five weeks—it may take that long before syphilis germs get into your bloodstream. So if your first blood test comes out negative, but you have reason to suspect you may have caught syphilis, return for another blood test a few weeks later.

The normal treatment for syphilis is penicillin. If you're allergic to penicillin, other antibiotics can be used just as effectively.

You're not cured, however, the moment you get the first shot. Several follow-up examinations, treatments, and blood tests are needed to make sure the disease is completely cured. It may take several months before all traces of syphilis infection disappear from your body.

GONORRHEA

Gonorrhea is not as deadly a disease as syphilis, but it's twice as dangerous. The clap—as gonorrhea is usually called—is much more common than syphilis, it's more contagious, and there are many more people who don't know they have it.

Unlike syphilis, gonorrhea infection is usually limited to the sex organs and the urinary system. But it can do plenty of damage there, and if it's not stopped, it can leave both men and women permanently sterile.

Gonorrhea germs live on the wet mucous lining of the urethra, the vagina, the anus, and the mouth. And the only way that gonorrhea can be transmitted from one person to another is during intercourse, anal intercourse, or oral sex, when these parts of the body are brought into direct contact with each other.

Gonorrhea infection develops much more rapidly than syphilis, and the course of the disease is different in men and women.

Men usually pick up gonorrhea through the urethral opening in the end of the penis. During intercourse with someone who's infected, the germs simply enter a man's penis and swim up the urethral tube.

Within three to seven days a man usually notices the first symptoms of infection. A thick, milky discharge starts oozing from the end of the penis. And there may be a painful burning sensation when he pisses.

These symptoms are usually enough to send a man running to the doctor. But there are some men, about one in five, who don't get these early signs of gonorrhea, or the symptoms are so mild they don't notice anything is wrong.

The disease, however, is highly contagious whether a man has painful symptoms or not. Any discharge from the penis, including semen, can easily infect a sexual partner since these fluids are teeming with gonorrhea germs.

If gonorrhea is not treated, the early symptoms will probably disappear in a few weeks. But the germs will continue to spread up through a man's urinary tract and reproductive system.

The infection can reach the bladder or invade the prostate gland and the seminal vesicles. Sometimes, but not always, this can cause painful inflammations in the internal tissues, and gonorrhea in the bladder can make it difficult or impossible to piss.

If the disease goes uncured or unnoticed for much more than a month, the germs will eventually travel all the way through a man's reproductive tubes until they reach the testicles. Here the infection not only causes painful swelling, but it starts doing permanent damage.

If gonorrhea is allowed to go on long enough, it can block the tiny tubes on top of the testicles completely, making it impossible for sperm to get from the testicles to the penis and thus leaving a man sterile.

However, it's very rare for the disease to progress that far. Somewhere along the line the infection will be extremely painful—either in the urethra, the bladder, the prostate, or the testicles. And most men are driven by the discomfort to get medical help before the disease can do much permanent damage.

With women it's a different story. Close to 80 percent of

all women infected with gonorrhea don't notice any painful symptoms in the first few weeks or even months. And many women discover they have gonorrhea only after it's done serious damage to their reproductive organs.

Gonorrhea infection usually starts in a woman's cervix. The germs multiply quickly inside the cervical opening, and within a few days pus starts to build up. But since the infection is painless and the cervix is deep inside the vagina, it's difficult for a woman to see or feel that anything is wrong.

Sometimes the infection produces a watery yellow discharge from the vagina, but it's not very heavy, and it frequently goes unnoticed.

Gonorrhea can also enter a woman's urethra. Here the infection can cause a burning sensation when she pisses, or it may spread to the bladder and make pissing frequent and painful.

If a woman notices any of these early signs, she's lucky. Most women don't feel any early symptoms and don't know they're infected at this point.

If the disease goes untreated for two or three months, the germs gradually work their way up from the cervix, through the uterus, and into the fallopian tubes. And gonorrhea in the fallopian tubes is very serious. The germs attack the inner walls of the fallopian tubes, scar tissue builds up, pus collects, and the tubes become blocked and swollen.

This may cause disruption in the menstrual periods, a fever, backaches, or severe pain throughout the entire abdominal area. The symptoms may be mild and linger over a period of several months, or they may strike a woman suddenly and painfully.

Even with antibiotics, which cure the gonorrhea infection, the scars on the fallopian tubes remain permanently. And if enough scar tissue has built up to block both tubes, a woman is left completely sterile. This happens frequently enough to be a real danger.

Whether the symptoms of gonorrhea are mild or painful, the disease is always contagious. And an infected woman can spread gonorrhea to anyone she has intercourse with.

The discharge that comes out of the vagina during the early stages of gonorrhea is also highly contagious, and it can spread the infection around the vaginal lips or down into the anus.

As many as half of all women who have gonorrhea in the vagina also have it in the rectum. Anal gonorrhea usually doesn't produce any obvious symptoms, and it can easily go unnoticed and uncured long after the disease has been cleared up in the reproductive organs.

A woman can also get gonorrhea in the rectum from having anal intercourse with an infected man. And male homosexuals have a high rate of anal gonorrhea, largely because the early signs aren't noticed, and the disease gets spread from partner to partner unknowingly.

It's also possible to get gonorrhea of the mouth. This is usually picked up by kissing or sucking the sex organs of an infected partner. Catching gonorrhea by mouth-to-mouth kissing is unlikely—and some doctors say almost impossible.

But gonorrhea of the mouth or rectum is just as dangerous as gonorrhea of the sexual organs. If left uncured for a long time, it can get into the bloodstream and cause serious damage to internal organs just like syphilis.

What this means is that all women who go for a gonorrhea test should have not only the genitals checked but also the anus. Male homosexuals should also get checked for anal gonorrhea. And everybody, male and female, who has had oral sex should have the mouth checked for infection.

Doctors will rarely if ever suggest this procedure. They're evidently more worried about offending you than they are about curing you. So you have to take the initiative if you want to get it cleared up. Insist on a thorough checkup. After all, it's your body.

At present there is no reliable blood test for gonorrhea like there is for syphilis. The only dependable way to diagnose gonorrhea is to take some fluid from the infected area and examine it.

In men this is done by inserting a cotton swab into the urethral opening in the penis. In women a swab is inserted into the cervix. To check for oral and anal gonorrhea, a sample is taken from the throat and the rectum. It's a simple, painless procedure, and it takes only a minute.

Although this is the best test available, it's not infallible. And if you have reason to suspect you may have gonorrhea—even though the test comes out negative—you should have a second test made. At public health clinics the tests are free, so it won't cost anything but a little time.

The most common treatment for gonorrhea is penicillin—either injected or taken orally. If you're allergic to penicillin, other antibiotics can be used. But since gonorrhea is becoming increasingly resistant to antibiotics, a massive dose is necessary to knock the disease out.

Even with large doses, only 80 percent to 90 percent of all people are cured with their first shot. That means that out of every one hundred people treated for gonorrhea, ten to twenty will not be cured immediately. The painful symptoms may disappear for a while, but you can still have the disease, and you can still pass it on to somebody else.

So it's important for everybody to return for a follow-up examination a week or ten days after the first treatment. A second or third shot is frequently needed to cure gonorrhea. And you shouldn't have sex with anybody until you know for sure that the disease is completely cleared up.

A FEW FACTS TO REMEMBER

The more you know about VD, the easier it is to protect yourself. And protect your partner. Here are a few additional points to keep in mind.

- There is no guaranteed way to prevent catching VD if your sexual partner has it. If the man uses a condom during sexual intercourse, it will reduce the chances of his getting VD or giving it to his partner, but it won't eliminate the possibility completely. Condoms can break, fluids can leak out, and VD can be transmitted where a man's scrotum comes in contact with a woman's vaginal lips.
- Washing with soap and water after intercourse can help cut down the risk of infection. Soap and water will kill VD germs on contact.
- Douching after intercourse can also reduce the chances of

catching VD. A woman can't douche if she's using vaginal foam or a diaphragm for birth control, however, there's some evidence that the foam itself helps protect a woman against VD.

• Pissing after intercourse can also help. Gonorrhea germs swim up the urethra, and pissing immediately after intercourse can sometimes flush them out.

• You can get both syphilis and gonorrhea at the same time. In fact, they frequently travel together. When you go for a gonorrhea test, always have a blood test done for syphilis too. When you go for a syphilis test, always have a sample taken for gonorrhea.

• Because 80 percent of women don't show any signs of gonorrhea, all sexually active women should have a gonorrhea test at least once a year. Every time a woman has a pelvic exam, she should also be examined for VD.

• Women should also remember to always have the anus checked for gonorrhea. And if they've had oral sex, they should have the mouth checked too.

• Both syphilis and gonorrhea can be passed on to an unborn child. Pregnant women should always make sure to get a complete VD checkup.

• Your body does not build up any immunity to either syphilis or gonorrhea. This means that you can catch VD, get cured, and catch it again.

• You cannot cure VD yourself. Don't even try. Taking penicillin pills or other antibiotics you have around in the medicine cabinet will not provide the massive doses you need to cure a case of VD. It may only make VD more difficult to diagnose. If you suspect that something is wrong, go to a doctor or clinic as soon as you can.

• If you find out you have VD, it's your responsibility to tell everyone you've had sex with so they can go for a checkup too. If you don't, they may never find out they have VD until it's done serious damage.

• If you're being treated for VD, don't have sex with anybody until it's completely cleared up. Even while you're being treated it's possible to infect your partner. So wait. It may take several weeks to get rid of gonorrhea and several months for syphilis.

WHERE TO GET VD TESTS AND TREATMENT

In most places there's no problem about minors getting treated for VD without their parents' consent. Since the spread of VD has reached such epidemic proportions, forty-six states and the District of Columbia have now made special exceptions to their health laws that allow minors to get confidential treatment for VD on their own consent.

However, in Iowa you have to be sixteen or over to get help on your own, and the law says you have to be fourteen or over in Idaho, New Hampshire, North Dakota, and Washington. If you're under the specified age, then you might have to fake it with some doctors and clinics.

In Wisconsin and Wyoming there is no provision for minors getting any kind of medical help without their parents' permission. And in Nebraska and Hawaii the law requires doctors to inform the parents of any minor who actually has VD. In those states you'll have to hunt around for a friendly doctor or a youth-oriented free clinic if you want to keep your sex life private.

In all the other states minors have the legal right to medical help for VD without involving their parents. You can get treated by a private doctor or a public clinic.

All doctors are required by law to report the name of every person who has VD to the local public health department. The reason for this is so that public health officials can track down the sexual partners of the infected person and bring them in for a VD exam. However, doctors ignore the law whenever it suits their convenience. Private doctors treating private patients in their own office rarely, if ever, report VD to the public health department. They don't want to lose a paying patient.

In public VD clinics, however, it's a different story. If your test shows you have syphilis or gonorrhea, a VD worker will ask you to name every person you've had sex with who could possibly have picked up the disease. If you refuse, they'll insist and hassle you.

Giving information on your sexual partners to a VD worker presents special problems. If you refuse, your partners may never get help. If you cooperate, you may be getting people in trouble.

VD workers will attempt to track down any people you name. They claim that they have all kinds of special methods for contacting young people without ever letting the parents know. But let's face it, when a VD worker comes around to a school or calls up at home, parents are going to get suspicious.

If you do give anybody's name as a sexual contact, try to get in touch with them first yourself and bring them down to the VD clinic, or have them call the VD worker. That will eliminate the possibility of the VD worker getting them in trouble accidentally.

If you go to a private doctor or a free clinic where there's no hassle, then it's your responsibility to contact everybody you've slept with who could also be infected. Remember, if you don't, they'll just be passing the disease around, and it's liable to come back to you again.

VD is a simple problem to diagnose and treat, and you can get help from any of the following:

Private doctors. They're expensive, but usually discreet. You'll have to insist on a thorough examination, since most private doctors are embarrassed about suggesting the possibility of oral or anal infection. All doctors are listed in the phone book under "Physicians."

Public health facilities. Every city has a public hospital that can handle VD. Larger cities have special VD clinics in neighborhood health centers. VD tests and treatment are free, but you have to wait in line. Call your local health department to find out where.

Free clinics and women's health centers. These are set up to help young people, and they're the least hassle. Check your local underground paper for ads, or look in the yellow pages under "Clinics."

Hotlines. Most youth-oriented hotlines will be able to tell you where to go for a VD test. In some cities there are special VD hotlines run by the public health department. Check the phone book or the last chapter of this book.

Planned Parenthood. Some centers give women VD tests and treatment. Call them; if they don't offer this service, maybe they can suggest a good place that does.

Planned Parenthood centers across the country can be found in the last chapter of this book, as well as a list of free clinics, women's centers, and public health facilities that diagnose and treat VD.

14

SEX AND THE LAW

The United States has more laws about sex than any other country in the world.

Most of these laws were written one hundred or two hundred years ago and haven't been changed much since. In general, they are based on the belief that the only legitimate purpose of sex is for married couples to have children.

So every other kind of sexual activity has been made illegal. All sex between unmarried men and women is outlawed. Homosexuality is a crime. And in many states even married couples aren't allowed to have oral or anal sex.

In addition, minors are subject to all kinds of special restrictions. Everything connected with sex—from going to the movies to getting married—is regulated by law. And in many states there are legal obstacles to minors getting birth control, abortion, or other health care that a sexually active person needs.

Not only does the law attempt to control every aspect of

a minor's sexual behavior, but at the same time the law also denies minors any rights—even over their own bodies.

As far as the law is concerned, minors are not independent people. They are considered property of their parents, and parental permission is required for just about everything.

The exact age at which you stop being a minor depends on where you live. In some states eighteen-year-olds have full legal rights, but in other states you have to be nineteen, twenty, or twenty-one before you can do what you want.

In the meantime, the law discriminates against you as long as you're a minor. And you can run into all kinds of hassles just because you're underage.

PERSONAL SEX LAWS

For all practical purposes, it's illegal for unmarried minors to have sex. The law may not say so exactly, but a dozen different laws in every state make anything besides kissing a crime.

In addition, there are a host of laws designed to protect minors from being morally corrupted by sex. Of course there's very little difference between being protected and being punished, and the way most of these laws work is simply to prohibit a minor from having sex at all.

For example, in every state the age at which an unmarried woman is considered old enough to have intercourse is set by law. This is called the Age of Consent, and as you can see from the accompanying chart, it varies from state to state depending on the whim of local lawmakers. In Louisiana and Tennessee a twelve-year-old girl is mature enough to make up her own mind about sex, but in California and Wisconsin you have to be eighteen.

The Age of Consent laws are intended to protect the chastity of young women and any man who has intercourse with a woman under the legal age is guilty of statutory rape. It doesn't matter how willing the woman is or how much she wants to have sex. In the eyes of the law she is too young to know what she's doing and the man who has sex with her is guilty of a serious crime.

AGE OF CONSENT

Until a female reaches the age shown below, she is considered too young to know what she's doing, and any male who has sexual intercourse with her may be guilty of statutory rape.

Alabama	16	Montana	18
Alaska	16	Nebraska	18
Arizona	18	Nevada	16
Arkansas	16	New Hampshire	16
California	18	New Jersey	16
Colorado	18	New Mexico	16
Connecticut	16	New York	17
Delaware	18*	North Carolina	16
District of Columbia	16	North Dakota	18
Florida	18	Ohio	16
Georgia	14	Oklahoma	16†
Hawaii	16	Oregon	16
Idaho	18	Pennsylvania	16
Illinois	16	Rhode Island	16
Indiana	16	South Carolina	16
Iowa	16	South Dakota	18
Kansas	18	Tennessee	12
Kentucky	18	Texas	18
Louisiana	12	Utah	18
Maine	14	Vermont	16
Maryland	16	Virginia	16
Massachusetts	18	Washington	18
Michigan	16	West Virginia	16
Minnesota	18	Wisconsin	18
Mississippi	18	Wyoming	18
Missouri	16		

* In Delaware the age of consent is actually seven years old, but any male who has intercourse with a female under eighteen can get seven years in jail.

† In Oklahoma the age of consent is sixteen, but it's still considered rape to take the virginity of a female between the ages of sixteen and eighteen.

The penalties for statutory rape vary widely from state to state, but there is usually a sliding scale depending on the age of the male as well as the age of the female. If the male is under the age of eighteen, the penalties are much less severe than if he is over twenty-one. But in some states even a minor can get twenty years just for sleeping with his girlfriend.

Obviously the statutory rape laws aren't enforced very often, or else half the young men in this country would be in jail. But if an underage female or her parents make a complaint, then the police are required to take action.

Once a woman reaches the Age of Consent, her sexual partner is no longer guilty of statutory rape. But now both the man and woman can be busted for a number of other crimes, including fornication, adultery, sodomy, and a variety of morals charges.

Fornication is the crime of fucking when you're not married. Most states have fornication laws, and most men and women are guilty of breaking them. This is a catchall law that can be applied to anyone regardless of age. Two sixty-year-olds who aren't married and have sex with each other can be busted for fornication. It's not very likely, but it's legally possible.

Adultery is usually defined as the crime married people commit when they have sex with someone besides their husband or wife. But in many states adultery laws apply to unmarried people as well. As long as one of the sexual partners is married, you can both be busted for adultery.

Sodomy is perhaps the broadest of all antisex laws. In most states the sodomy laws prohibit any form of "unnatural intercourse"—that is, any contact between the mouth and penis, the mouth and vagina, or the penis and the anus.

Although these laws were designed to prohibit homosexuality, they make almost everything illegal besides face-to-face intercourse. Under the sodomy laws not only homosexuals but also single men and women and even married couples have been prosecuted for having oral sex and anal intercourse.

And just in case you should think up some clever way to have sex that doesn't break any of the laws already mentioned, you should remember that minors can always be busted on a dozen other charges like "immoral behavior" or "sexual misconduct." These laws are so vague in most states that they include almost any kind of touching or stroking. In effect, these laws make it illegal for any minor, under or over the Age of Consent, to have any kind of sex.

And not only the law but law enforcement as well tends to discriminate against minors. The laws in this country make almost everybody a "sex criminal," but young people get busted much more frequently than adults. Every year more than 13,000 minors are arrested for sex offenses, and that doesn't include real crimes like rape or prostitution.

The penalties for sex offenses are usually mild, provided that both partners are minors and both wanted to have sex. But minors under the age of sixteen are classified as juveniles, and juveniles can always be sent to reform school "for their own good" or because they "need supervision." In fact, in a state like Connecticut, a juvenile can be locked up until the age of eighteen simply for being "in danger of becoming morally corrupted."

This doesn't mean everybody should get uptight about sex. But minors do have to be careful about their privacy. The only way these sex laws can be enforced is if you get caught by parents or police. Parents tend to get upset when they discover their daughter having sex, and cops love to bust young people in parked cars.

PARENTS, MARRIAGE, AND EMANCIPATION

As long as you're under eighteen, you're subject to your parents' authority. And parents are usually the biggest problem any minor has with sex.

Parents who don't want their kids to have sex can make life very difficult. For one thing, parental permission is required for everything from medical care to marriage. In addition, parents can bring a variety of legal charges against a man who is having sex with their daughter, especially if the man is over twenty-one.

If you should decide to run away, parents can always have you picked up and brought back. Usually the police won't bother with males over the age of sixteen, but any female can be prevented from leaving home until the age of eighteen. Every year more than 200,000 minors are arrested for running away.

The only legal way for a minor to escape parental authority is to become emancipated—and you usually need your parents' cooperation for that too. Emancipation is a legal term that means a minor is independent and living on his own.

Although there are no uniform standards from state to state, a minor would have to be at least sixteen, self-supporting, and living outside the family in order to be considered emancipated. Then you have the right, in most states, to take care of yourself medically and morally.

But unless you graduate from high school very early and have a steady job, this isn't a very realistic alternative for most people under eighteen. However, you can always claim to be emancipated when you need medical care or birth control. If you look old enough, you can frequently get away with it.

When it comes to getting married, the law is very specific. Every state has both a minimum age for getting married on your own and a minimum age for getting married with parental consent. The exact ages, state by state, are shown on the accompanying marriage chart.

Parents cannot force you to get married, but they can force you to stay single as long as you're a minor. Until you reach the minimum age for marrying without parental consent, which is usually eighteen for females and twenty-one for males, it's impossible to get a marriage license on your own.

Should you somehow succeed in getting married by lying about your age, parents can always take legal action to have the marriage dissolved—especially if the woman is below the Age of Consent in your state.

And if a couple decide to travel to another state where the age is lower, they face a host of possible legal problems. In the first place, the man can be charged with "abduction"—the crime of stealing an underage woman away from her parents. It makes no difference if the female is a willing partner or not, because it is the parents who bring charges against the man for stealing their daughter.

Abduction laws vary from state to state, but they can usually be applied whenever the female is under the legal minimum

MARRIAGE LAWS

Every state sets the minimum age for getting married with and without parental consent. To check these laws, call your local marriage license bureau.

	With Parental Consent		Without Parental Consent	
	Male	Female	Male	Female
Alabama	17	14	21	18
Alaska	18*	16*	19	18
Arizona	18*	16*	18†	18
Arkansas	18*	16*	21	18
California	18	16	21	18
Colorado	16*	16*	21	18
Connecticut	16*	16*	18†	18†
Delaware	18*	16*	18†	18†
District of Columbia	18	16	21	18
Florida	18*	16*	21	21
Georgia	18*	16*	19	19
Hawaii	18*	16*	20	18
Idaho	18*	16*	21	18
Illinois	18*	16*	21	18
Indiana	18*	16*	21	18
Iowa	18*	16*	21	18
Kansas	18*	18*	21	18
Kentucky	18*	16*	18	18
Louisiana	18*	16*	21	21
Maine	16*	16*	18†	18
Maryland	18*	16*	21	18
Massachusetts	18*	16*	18	18
Michigan	18	16*	18	18

Minnesota	18	16	21	18
Mississippi	17*	15*	21	18
Missouri	15*	15*	21	18
Montana	18	16	21	18
Nebraska	18*	16*	21	21
Nevada	18*	16*	18†	18
New Hampshire	14	13	20	18
New Jersey	18*	16*	18	18
New Mexico	18*	16*	21	18
New York	16	14	21	18
North Carolina	16	16*	18	18
North Dakota	18	15	18†	18
Ohio	18*	16*	21	21
Oklahoma	18*	15*	21	18
Oregon	18	15	21	18
Pennsylvania	16*	16*	21	21
Rhode Island	18*	16*	21	21
South Carolina	16*	14*	18	18
South Dakota	18	16*	18†	18†
Tennessee	16*	16*	18	18
Texas	16	14	19	18
Utah	16	14	21	18
Vermont	18*	16*	18†	18
Virginia	18*	16*	18†	18†
Washington	17*	17*	18	18
West Virginia	18*	16*	18†	18†
Wisconsin	18	16	18†	18†
Wyoming	18	16	18†	18†

* Under certain circumstances, like pregnancy or childbirth, younger people may be married with parental consent and special permission of the court.

† Although there are old laws on the books that set a higher minimum age for marrying without parental consent, this state has recently granted eighteen-year-olds full legal rights.

age for marrying without her parents' consent. And if your state doesn't have an abduction law, a woman under the age of eighteen can always be arrested for running away.

In addition, many states do not recognize marriages contracted by minors in another state for the specific purpose of avoiding your own state's minimum-age law.

If you're not interested in getting married but decide to move in with your lover, then you face another set of legal obstacles.

Most states have laws against "lewd cohabitation" that make it illegal for two people of the opposite sex to live together without being married. These laws are rarely enforced against adults, but they can always be enforced against minors if the parents complain to the police.

And if the female of the couple happens to be under the Age of Consent—which is eighteen in Massachusetts, Wisconsin, and California—the male can always be charged with a number of other crimes like statutory rape.

All in all, minors are at the mercy of their parents until they reach the age of eighteen. You can't run away, move out, or get married without their permission. And they have the legal right to interfere with your sexual relationship if they don't approve.

MEDICAL CARE FOR MINORS

There is no problem about minors getting medical care when they have their parents' consent. However, when it comes to getting medical care on your own—especially medical care related to sex—there are all kinds of restrictions.

To begin with, minors are under the legal care and custody of their parents, and no one may tamper with a minor's health without parental consent. This means that a doctor who treats a minor without any legal authorization is liable to a variety of charges brought by the parents.

For example, if a doctor prescribes birth-control pills for a woman under eighteen without her parents' permission, the parents could bring legal charges of malpractice and assault against the doctor. The doctor could even be accused of "contributing to the delinquency of a minor" for encouraging a woman to have sex before she's married.

Charges like these are very rare, but the legal possibility of angry parents going to court has been enough to keep many doctors from treating minors on their own. Doctors, after all, are very careful about protecting themselves and their medical licenses.

In addition, many states have passed specific laws restricting birth control and abortion for minors without parental consent. The purpose of these laws is to prevent minors from having sex as freely as adults.

Of course laws have never prevented anybody from fucking, but they have made it difficult for minors to get the medical care they need. As a result, minors have more venereal disease, more illegitimate babies, and more deaths from homemade abortions than any other age group.

In some states minors have been given limited rights to get certain medical care on their own. Married and emancipated minors can usually give their own consent. In some states female minors have the right to get their own medical care for pregnancy. And because of the venereal disease epidemic, most states have been forced to allow minors to get treated for VD without parental permission.

Despite these recent changes, there are still hundreds of restrictions on the books. And when it comes to something like birth control, many states have totally absurd and contradictory laws.

In New Jersey, for example, a minor has to be pregnant before she can legally get contraception. In California any minor can get an abortion on her own, but only married and emancipated minors can get birth control to prevent an accidental pregnancy.

In New York any minor may buy contraceptive foam and condoms from a drugstore at sixteen, but women have to be eighteen before they can get pills and other prescriptive birth control from a doctor.

These laws are so unfair—and so confusing—that they are frequently ignored. Free clinics and youth clinics, for example, were started in many cities for the specific purpose of giving minors medical care on their own. And organizations like

Planned Parenthood often overlook the stipulation of parental consent when a minor needs help.

In addition, private doctors can usually get around state laws if they want to. Most states have provisions in their health laws that allow doctors to treat a minor in an emergency or when the attempt to get parental consent would delay treatment and risk a minor's health.

So when you need medical care on your own, you can always insist it's an emergency. And it's important to remember that even when it's not legal for a doctor to treat a minor, it's never illegal for a minor to get treated. This means that if you lie about your age or claim to be married or emancipated, you're not breaking any law. The laws, in this case, apply only to doctors.

PREGNANCY AND PATERNITY

If you're under eighteen and unmarried, getting pregnant can present a lot of serious problems. Most of the problems are with parents, but state laws can create some hassle too.

No matter what you decide to do about your pregnancy, the law makes it difficult for you to act on your own. If you want to have an abortion, most states require women under eighteen to have parental permission.

If you decide not to have an abortion, you may face many more problems, including school, adoption, and possibly even your right to have a baby at all.

Suppose, for example, that you want to get married and have your baby, but your parents want you to have an abortion and finish school. Even if you're pregnant, you can't get married without your parents' approval if you're still underage. And your parents can arrange an abortion even if you don't want one.

There have been many cases exactly like this in the last several years. Sometimes a minor can succeed in having her child; other times she is forced by her parents or the courts to have an abortion. Minors do not have any absolute rights, not even the right to determine when they will give birth.

One recent and very real example of this problem involved a sixteen-year-old girl in Maryland. The girl's parents refused permission for her to marry her boyfriend and insisted on an abortion. The night before the operation was to be performed, the young couple ran away.

They were both arrested and thrown in jail. A local judge ruled that the girl was "a person in need of supervision" and ordered her to be kept in jail until she obeyed her parents and had an abortion. Fortunately the girl got a lawyer, who appealed her case to a higher court and eventually won her the right to bear the child she wanted.

But most cases do not end so happily. If you should ever find yourself in this particular conflict with your parents, you'll definitely need legal help. Lawyers can frequently stall such a case until it's too late to have an abortion, and you get what you want by default.

Meanwhile, if you're pregnant, you can have many problems with school. In principle, the state has an obligation to provide public education for everyone until the age of eighteen, but thousands of young women have been thrown out of school for being pregnant. School administrators in many places seem to think that a pregnant woman will be such a bad example that she will morally corrupt all the other students and make education impossible.

The attitudes and even the laws about pregnant women in school vary from state to state and town to town. In Ohio, for example, the courts have upheld the right of school administrators to expel pregnant students. But in New York pregnant students can stay in their neighborhood school or go to a special school for pregnant women if they want.

After you've had your baby, you might face other kinds of legal problems. If your parents don't want you to keep the child, you might be forced to give it up. If you've been busted for something like drugs, the courts can take the child away from you for being an "unfit mother."

Even if you decide yourself to give a baby up for adoption, it's important to get legal help. Adoption laws get very complicated, and if you ever change your mind in the future and want your child back, you would have all kinds of legal hassle.

Another side to the problem of pregnancy is paternity, or fatherhood. The father, even if he's a minor, is legally and financially responsible for his child from the moment pregnancy begins.

This means that a man under eighteen can be held responsible for all expenses involved in pregnancy, birth, and child care. And the father's obligations continue until his child is eighteen, regardless of whether the child is legitimate or illegitimate.

Paternity lawsuits, in which the young father is sued for child support, are usually started by a pregnant woman or her parents. And they're nothing to be taken lightly. However, if the man has reason to doubt he is really the father of the child, or if he thinks he's being framed, there are several things he can do.

First of all, blood tests can prove that a man is definitely not the father of a child if his blood and the child's do not match up. If they do match, it still doesn't prove a man definitely is the father.

Second, if a man can prove to a court that there is good reason to suspect he is not the father—for example, if he can show that several other men were having sex with the same woman at the same time—then he may still get out of it.

Pregnancy, of course, does not have to involve all these problems for either a woman or a man. But it can, and it's good to keep them in mind. And if you do have problems, you're going to need legal help. You have a much better chance of protecting yourself if you have a lawyer on your side.

PORNOGRAPHY AND CENSORSHIP

Society's attitude toward sex and minors is completely unrealistic. And nowhere is this more obvious than in the laws against obscenity and pornography.

Pornography is always a hard thing to define, since different people have different standards. But according to most laws, any book, magazine, or movie whose only purpose is to sexually stimulate the audience is prohibited. In other words, sex in itself and for its own pleasure is considered obscene and illegal.

Nevertheless, there has been a flood of pornographic material produced in the last few years, and it's available in every major city. The Supreme Court has even ruled that adults have the right to own pornography and enjoy it in the privacy of their own home. But there is no such legal right for minors.

In fact, our society has an absolutely crazy fear that minors may see, hear, or read anything about sex. Almost all censorship laws are based on the notion of "protecting children." And every state has a host of laws that forbid selling sexy books or pictures to minors.

New York, for example, has a law against selling minors any literature that depicts "sexual excitement or sexual arousal." Under this law everything from *Playboy* to Shakespeare would be illegal until you're twenty-one.

In Texas the law says that minors under eighteen may not see any material that shows "sexual parts of the human body without clothing—including the buttocks and a woman's breasts below the top of the nipple." So it would be illegal in Texas, as in many other states, for a married seventeen-year-old to see a picture of the female breast.

The most glaring example of this absurd attitude toward sex is the rating code of the Motion Picture Association of America. This code, which is made up by film producers and theater owners, defines what movies a minor may or may not see.

According to the rating system, persons under seventeen are not admitted to R movies without a parent or guardian. And no one under seventeen (or eighteen in some states) is admitted to an X-rated movie.

Films that carry an X or R rating are not considered obscene or pornographic according to state laws. They're just regular movies with a little nudity or some "dirty" language. But minors are prevented from seeing them, because minors aren't supposed to be exposed to any kind of sex at all.

The theory behind all these censorship laws is that seeing a naked human body or being sexually aroused will automatically lead a person to a life of immorality, vice, and crime.

However, every scientific study ever made, including the study done by the President's Commission on Obscenity and Pornography, indicates just the opposite. It is usually the sex criminal, the pervert, and the rapist who have had the least exposure to pornography. They attack other people precisely because they do not have any other outlet like books, magazines, or movies. In a country like Denmark, which legalized all forms of pornography, sex crimes have been cut in half.

Pornography does have the effect of temporarily stimulating most people. It may even serve to encourage masturbation. But there's nothing wrong with masturbation, and seeing too much pornography does not lead to crime, it only leads to boredom.

Censorship laws, however, are not based on facts, they're based on fears. They're an attempt to control what other people may see or do or think. And in addition to prohibiting sex, censorship laws are often used to stifle free speech.

Underground newspapers and high school reading lists are frequently censored by puritanical authorities who suppress whatever they don't like on the grounds of obscenity or pornography. Here, as in so many other things, minors are denied their basic human rights in the name of morality.

WHERE TO GET LEGAL HELP

There are dozens of reasons why a minor might need some kind of legal information or assistance.

If you want to get married or leave home or have an abortion, you may need to check your state laws. If you get caught fucking on a public beach or get thrown out of school for using obscene language, then you'll probably need a lawyer to defend you.

And getting legal help is not as difficult as it sounds. Private lawyers, like private doctors, are usually expensive. But there are many places where you can get free legal information and advice if you know where to look.

Public services. Almost every city has some kind of public legal-assistance agency designed to help people who can't afford private lawyers. Depending on where you live, this agency might be called the Public Defenders Office, Community Legal Service, Neighborhood Legal Assistance, Legal Aid Society, or something else. You can usually find these agencies in the phone book along with other government services. However, like most public services, they are usually understaffed and overworked and may not have time to provide the best-quality help.

Civil Liberties Union. This is a national organization devoted to protecting the constitutional rights of every citizen. They have done a lot of work with minors, especially in the field of students' rights. And although they don't handle every kind of legal problem, they can always offer good advice and refer you to another agency for further help.

There are chapters of the Civil Liberties Union in almost every state, and they can be found in the phone book under American Civil Liberties Union or under state listings like Alabama Civil Liberties Union.

National Lawyers Guild. This is a private organization of lawyers who offer their services to people who can't find or afford other lawyers. They are usually more liberal, more sympathetic, and more helpful than public agencies, and they may be more familiar with the legal problems of minors.

There are twenty-six chapters of the National Lawyers Guild in cities across the country. Check your local phone book.

Hotlines. There are many legal switchboards across the country that are staffed by law students and volunteer lawyers. These switchboards will give you information and advice over the phone or refer you to other organizations for specific help.

In addition, many general hotlines and free clinics also give legal assistance. In fact, many hotlines and clinics have special legal counselors to handle problems with the law. These services are usually the most sympathetic and the most helpful for minors.

Free clinics, hotlines, and private agencies that offer legal help and advice are listed in the last chapter of this book.

15

SEX AND DRUGS

People take drugs for lots of different reasons—for kicks, for curiosity, for the fun of being high. And one of the reasons some people use drugs is to increase the physical pleasure of sex.

There are all kinds of myths about the sexual powers of drugs. Some drugs are supposed to turn you into a sexual superman; others are supposed to make sex completely impossible. Most of these stories, however, are not very reliable.

In the first place, drugs don't affect your genitals; they work on your brain and your nervous system. That means any drug that gets you high will change your total mental, physical, and emotional state—not just your sex drive.

Some drugs can lower your inhibitions, relax your muscles, and increase your awareness of your own body. As a result, everything you do—including sex—may seem more pleasurable. But the same drug might make another person tense, nauseous, and unreceptive to sex.

Drugs, after all, are chemicals that react differently in every person's body. And since there's such a wide variety of reactions to any single drug, it's very difficult to say exactly how somebody is going to respond physically, psychologically, or sexually.

How a drug affects you depends on a great many things, like your body chemistry, your mood, and your past experience with the drug. Even your expectations can influence how you respond to a particular drug.

There's also a great deal of difference between using drugs occasionally and taking them every day. Drugs aren't something your body naturally needs, like sex. And getting stoned all the time only fucks you up—mentally as well as physically.

While certain drugs may enhance your physical sensations, the pleasure of sex usually depends more on how you feel about your sex partner than on what drugs you put into your body.

GRASS AND HASH

Marijuana is used by millions of people. It's relatively safe, cheap, and easy to get.

Getting high on grass usually intensifies whatever you're experiencing at the moment. If you're feeling depressed or frightened, grass just might make it worse. If you're in a good mood, grass will probably make it even better. In fact, most people find getting high on grass is pleasant and amusing.

Grass affects your head—it distorts reality a little bit. It also increases your awareness, making you pick up on a hundred little details about yourself and the outside world that you don't ordinarily notice.

Actually grass is a mild hallucinogenic drug. If you smoke enough, you can have visual hallucinations and experience dreamlike feelings and sounds. And everybody who's into drugs is familiar with the experience of having a very profound insight while you're stoned, only to find that it's a pretty stupid idea the next day—that is, if you can remember it at all.

Grass also affects your body. It makes you feel relaxed and increases physical sensitivity. Colors and sounds become richer, and your sense of touch is intensified.

All this usually makes sex feel especially good when you're

high. And besides, the drug usually lowers inhibitions, making you feel freer and more open about sex.

And since you tend to get hung up on things when you're stoned, sex can be very sensual and engrossing. You may really get into your partner's body and the pleasure of your own body on grass. And having an orgasm may seem more intense than usual.

Hashish, which is the compressed resin of the marijuana plant, is usually stronger than grass. While a grass high is light and giggly, being stoned on hash is usually a heavier, more sluggish trip.

But basically the effects of the two drugs are the same. Hash disorients your head and produces the same increased sensitivity to your body and your surroundings.

The chemical property in both grass and hash that gets you high is called THC or tetrahydrocannabinol. THC can be synthesized, and although it's very rare, it can sometimes be found in pill form.

THC is a convenient way to get high for people who don't like to smoke. But the same problem exists with THC that exists with all other pills—you can never be sure of what you're taking. In fact, many drug people think that THC isn't available at all anymore and that whatever you buy is just a worthless or poisonous substitute.

It's important to remember that not everybody responds the same way to grass and hash. Some people say grass has no effect on them at all, and other people don't like the kind of sensations these drugs produce. And there are some people who like to get high but don't like to have sex while they're stoned because they feel too lazy or distracted.

But whatever your reactions may be, grass is pretty safe. You can control how high you get by how much you smoke. And it's impossible to overdose. Grass is not physically addictive, and it doesn't lead to anything except hunger pangs.

ALCOHOL

Alcohol is used so widely in this country that most people don't even think of it as a drug. But alcohol is a drug, and it can put your head, as well as your body, through all kinds of changes.

Alcohol is a strong depressant that works directly on your brain. It interferes with physical coordination and control; it makes it difficult to think in an organized and logical fashion; and it lowers your normal inhibitions.

Getting high on alcohol gives most people a pleasant light-headed sensation. It slows down your body and makes everything a little fuzzy. And despite the fact that alcohol is a depressant, it can also make you feel more talkative and energetic for a while.

That's why alcohol is so popular in social situations—it makes people feel both relaxed and lively. Unfortunately alcohol can also be an antisocial drug. A lot of anger and violence break out because people are drunk.

Many people think that alcohol also increases your sex drive. But that's not really true. It lowers your inhibitions and makes you feel less self-conscious. That can make it easier for sex to come out, but it doesn't really change your sexual appetites.

In fact, drinking too much interferes with sex—and everything else. Alcohol eventually makes you sluggish and numb. A man can have difficulty getting an erection when he's drunk, and a woman can have trouble reaching orgasm. Too much alcohol makes you feel more like going to sleep than having sex.

Drinking is an accepted and approved part of our culture, but you have to be smart about alcohol—just like any other drug. Getting high is fun, but getting stoned drunk will only make you sick.

PSYCHEDELICS

When it comes to the major psychedelic drugs like LSD and mescaline, it's very difficult to give an accurate description of their sexual side effects. These drugs radically distort all of your physical and emotional perceptions, and what you experience when you're high may have little or nothing to do with normal reality.

The oldest of all the psychedelic drugs is peyote, the

mushroom-shaped bud of a cactus plant. It has been eaten since the time of the Aztec Indians to induce magical visions. Today peyote is scarce, but its active ingredient, mescaline, has been synthesized and is sold in pill or powder form.

There are many varieties of mescaline around, and your experience with the drug can depend entirely on the kind of mescaline you take—whether it's organic or synthetic, whether it's pure or laced with speed.

If you swallow an average dose of mescaline, the effect of the drug will last about eight hours, and it can be a physically exhausting experience. Your first reaction is liable to be nausea or even vomiting. But for most people this passes within an hour and the hallucinogenic high begins.

Mescaline affects all your senses. Colors look brighter and sharper, and you may experience flickering vision, where everything appears to be moving under a strobe light. Time slows down, your sense of space changes, and you may think you are ten feet tall one minute and a dwarf the next.

Having sex when you're high can be a very intense experience—all the physical and emotional sensations of sex become magnified. Your body is likely to feel weightless and extremely sensual. At times it may even feel like different parts of your body aren't attached to the rest of you.

There's not much physical danger in taking pure mescaline, but it does leave you feeling totally wasted the next day. However, if you inhale the powdered drug through your nose instead of swallowing it, you will have a lighter trip that doesn't last as long and doesn't leave you quite as exhausted.

LSD, on the other hand, does involve certain dangers because it's highly unpredictable. Unlike grass, mescaline, or other psychedelic drugs, acid does not rely on the things you see or hear to produce its distortions and hallucinations. It creates its own visions totally independent of external reality.

Acid seems to work by breaking down certain psychological barriers, so that a person is bombarded with sensations from the outside world and from the subconscious mind at the same time. And often you can't tell the difference between them.

For some people acid is a revealing and exciting experience. For others it can be extremely frightening. A person who isn't used to the drug will usually feel overwhelmed by it and go through extremes of mood and emotion during the long trip.

Fucking on acid can be very dramatic—you may experience all kinds of unusual physical sensations. But it's sometimes impossible to distinguish between what's really happening and what you're hallucinating.

The trouble with acid is that it's impossible to control your own trip. You don't direct the drug—it directs you. And while sex may be fantastically pleasurable, this is not the kind of drug that people should take just for sexual novelty. You have to know what you're doing when you use acid.

UPS AND DOWNS

Tranquilizers and barbiturates, commonly called downs, are drugs that depress the central nervous system. Medically they're used to relieve tension and induce sleep. But many people also take downs because they produce a quiet, euphoric kind of high.

Tranquilizers are relatively mild drugs. There are hundreds of commercial brands manufactured, but the most well known on the underground market are probably Librium, Miltown, and Equanil.

Barbiturates are much stronger drugs than tranquilizers, and they're used as sleeping pills. Amytal, Nembutal, Seconal, and Tuinal are some of the better-known commercial barbiturates.

The effect of these drugs is felt throughout the entire body as muscles relax and tension disappears. If you're feeling tired to begin with, downs may only put you to sleep. If you're not sleepy, you get a pleasant, light-headed kind of feeling.

In fact, being stoned on downs is similar to being drunk on alcohol. Your reflexes are slowed, your reactions are dulled, and your speech may get slurred.

For many people downs don't produce any special sexual effect. But other people find that their body is more relaxed and sensual when they're high, and as a result, sex feels much better.

While one or two downs may loosen people up, too many

downs can interfere with sexual response. This means a man may have trouble keeping his erection, and a woman may find it hard to reach orgasm. But most people who take downs are so relaxed they don't care.

Downs are good for sex only if you take them occasionally in moderate amounts. It's important to realize that downs are addictive when they're taken steadily, and a barbiturate addict doesn't get much pleasure from sex or anything else.

In addition to getting addicted, it's also possible to overdose on downs. Taking too many barbiturates can kill you. Mixing them with alcohol is also dangerous because alcohol increases their strength.

Perhaps the most popular of all barbiturates is methaqualone, which is manufactured under a variety of brand names like Quaalude, Sopor, and Optimil. Methaqualone became widely popular because it was supposed to be an aphrodisiac and because the manufacturers claimed it wasn't addictive.

Unfortunately methaqualone is not an aphrodisiac, and like all other barbiturates, it is addictive. What's more, trying to withdraw from this drug is even harder than getting off a heroin habit, because methaqualone can produce fatal convulsions if a regular user stops taking it too suddenly.

Amphetamines, or ups, have the opposite effect of barbiturates. They stimulate the central nervous system, so instead of slowing you down, they speed you up.

Of the various commercial brands of mild amphetamines, Benzedrine and Dexedrine are probably most well known. Medically they're used as stimulants or diet pills, since they relieve fatigue and supress your appetite. They're also widely used by students who have to stay awake and concentrate for long periods of time.

The most powerful form of amphetamine is Methedrine—commonly called speed. It's usually sold as a powder that can be injected or inhaled. Shooting Methedrine has an effect about a thousand times stronger than swallowing a couple of Dexedrine, and it's much more dangerous too. Inhaling the stuff is safer, although it's not so great for the inside of your nose.

Getting high on any kind of amphetamine affects you mentally as well as physically. Your brain buzzes along at ninety miles an hour while your body feels tremendously energetic. All your muscles become tense, and you may feel jittery and excitable. Depending on what you like, this feeling can be very stimulating or very uncomfortable.

Sexual reactions to amphetamines also vary greatly from person to person. Many people find that amphetamines reduce their sexual appetite. Others think amphetamines make their body more sensitive and use these drugs just to increase the pleasure of sex.

Amphetamines certainly do give you more physical stamina. It's possible to fuck for hours when you're high on ups—and you may have to, since the drug can delay orgasm for both men and women.

Like barbiturates, the sexual side effects of amphetamines can depend on how often you take them. If you don't use ups very often, they may be stimulating. But people who take this drug all the time usually lose interest in sex completely.

And while amphetamines aren't supposed to be physically addictive, they are dangerous if you take them regularly. Long-term use of ups—especially Methedrine—eventually destroys your brain and your body.

NARCOTICS

Opium, heroin, and cocaine are probably the most well-known narcotics, although there are many others. Narcotics have the effect of numbing the senses, and except for cocaine, they're all addictive.

Opium comes from the poppy flower, grown in Asia and the Middle East. It's been smoked for centuries to produce a sleepy, euphoric kind of high. But it's hard to get in this country, and opium addicts are rare.

Sex on opium can be gentle and sensuous, because all your muscles are relaxed and your body feels very loose. But opium has a strong narcotic effect that can put you to sleep before you ever get around to having sex. And after sex you don't stand a chance of staying awake.

Heroin is probably the most widely used hard drug in this

country. Although it's derived from opium, heroin is much stronger, but it's greatly diluted before it's sold. Usually it's diluted with quinine or milk sugar, but sometimes it's cut with rat poison, which can kill you.

People who are used to taking heroin experience a mildly euphoric high when they shoot or snort this drug. Everyday problems and tensions disappear, and the body drifts into a drowsy state of well-being. But if you've never taken heroin before, it's liable to make you sick or just put you to sleep.

Heroin isn't a sex drug, and nobody really takes it for sex. In fact, junkies are often impotent. Sex can feel pleasant if you snort a little heroin through your nose, but at the same time you may have trouble reaching orgasm. And many people simply aren't interested in sex when they're high on this drug.

The problems involved in heroin have been well publicized, and everybody knows about them. You can never be sure what the drug is cut with, it's possible to overdose, and giving yourself any kind of injection is dangerous.

Besides, heroin is addictive, and long-term use of this drug destroys the body. People who snort heroin only occasionally have a much better chance of avoiding these traps than people who get into shooting, but it's still a very risky drug to mess around with.

There are many synthetic heroin substitutes, like methadone, which are sold in pill form. They aren't used as sexual turn-ons, and methadone addicts have even been known to complain of sexual impotence. If you don't have a heroin habit to begin with, these substitutes may make you nauseous instead of high.

Cocaine is another drug classified as a narcotic, although it has the opposite effect of other hard drugs. Cocaine is a stimulant, and it was one of the original ingredients in Coca-Cola until the government banned it.

When cocaine is inhaled or injected, it stimulates the nervous system the same way amphetamine does. Cocaine kills your appetite, increases your energy, and makes you feel very alert and elated.

Sexual reactions to cocaine depend very much on the individual. Many people experience a decrease in their sex drive, but others find that the drug enhances sex. Cocaine does increase strength and stamina, which can be positive qualities when it comes to sex.

Although it's not physically addictive, you can overdose on cocaine. And like all strong drugs, it's dangerous if you take it all the time.

INHALANTS

People inhale all kinds of stuff from burning tobacco to laughing gas in order to get high. Some of these things are fairly harmless, but others are extremely dangerous.

Inhaling airplane glue, for example, will give you a dizzy kind of feeling for a while. But it also gives you brain damage. Inhale enough of the stuff and you'll be permanently dizzy.

Freon, the gas from aerosol cans and sprays, is also inhaled for its euphoric effects. It produces a light-headed sensation, but it's very harmful to your lungs, and it can easily kill you.

Neither of these chemicals does anything for sex, and neither of them was ever intended for human consumption. If you like your body and want to stay alive, you should avoid them both.

Amyl nitrite, on the other hand, is an inhalant that's often used specifically for sex. Medically the drug was designed to relieve heart seizures by enlarging the blood vessels and speeding up the heart. But it can also intensify sexual pleasure.

Amyl nitrite comes in capsules, or poppers, which are broken and inhaled like smelling salts. Within a few seconds you can feel the effect of the drug. Your heart starts pounding, and you're liable to feel hot, flushed, and dizzy.

The effect of amyl nitrite lasts only a few minutes. But if you inhale a popper while you're having sex, the rush of the drug can immediately raise sexual excitement to the point of orgasm. And when you do come, it may feel longer and more powerful than normally.

In some places amyl nitrite is still available in any drugstore, but in most states it's sold by prescription only. And although it's a very powerful drug, it's not known to be dangerous provided it's used only occasionally.

BAD DOPE AND BUM TRIPS

Some of the drugs mentioned in this chapter can be legally obtained only with a doctor's prescription, others are illegal under any circumstances. And while the law never seemed to discourage anyone from experimenting with drugs, it should be kept in mind. For one thing, you can always be busted for possessing drugs.

But what's even more important, there's absolutely no protection for the person who buys illegal drugs. If you buy grass or hash, you can usually be sure of what you're getting. But most other drugs sold on city streets just aren't what the dealer claims.

For example, what's sold as "mescaline" is usually LSD or the waste products from making acid combined with some animal tranquilizers. This kind of chemical junk makes most people pretty sick.

Drugs that are sold in powder form, especially narcotics, are frequently stretched with dangerous stuff. And when you are lucky enough to get a pure drug, like acid, it's liable to be four or five times the dose anybody should take.

There are plenty of drugs that gain a reputation, like DMT, STP, and THC, that simply can't be bought anymore. What you get instead is some mixture of barbiturates, animal drugs, and acid—a combination that's designed to produce some very unpleasant surprises.

And new drugs come along all the time, drugs that turn out to destroy brain cells, rot your kidneys, or drive you crazy. But that's usually not discovered until a few thousand guinea pigs have wound up in emergency rooms.

Having sex when you're high can be a beautiful experience. But unless you know what you're doing and you know the drug is pure, it's not a good idea to just throw stuff into your system. Getting sick or poisoned isn't the best way to enjoy the pleasures of your body.

16

WHERE TO GET HELP

This is a state-by-state directory of services across the country that offer help to people under eighteen.

The services on this list can help you get birth control, pregnancy tests, VD tests, general medical care, abortions, or legal help. There are several types of facilities listed, and they include:

Free clinics. Medical clinics that are free or very inexpensive. Many free clinics are specifically set up to help young people. In addition to confidential medical care, free clinics often provide counseling for a variety of problems.

Women's health centers. These centers are set up to deal with the medical needs of women, especially when it comes to birth control and abortion. Some of the women's centers on this list are actual medical clinics; others are counseling and referral services.

Planned Parenthood. A national birth-control organization with clinics across the country. In addition to contraception, many Planned Parenthood centers offer other services for women, like pregnancy tests, VD tests, and abortion referral. Some Planned Parenthood centers have special teen clinics for women under eighteen.

Public health departments. Public health departments on this list run free or inexpensive clinics for birth control, pregnancy tests, VD tests, and other kinds of medical care. Also listed are public health department referral services that will direct you to a local clinic in your neighborhood.

Clergy Consultation Service on Abortion. A national organization that can help you find the best abortion facility in your area. Clergy Consultation workers can also make referrals for pregnancy tests, and they offer sympathetic counseling for young women who don't want to involve their parents.

Hotlines and counseling services. These are telephone services that can tell you where to go for medical or legal help. They will usually know which clinics in your town require parental consent for medical treatment and which clinics will help you on your own.

Many of the clinics and hotlines in this directory are set up to handle a wide variety of problems. Some are into drug emergencies, some are into psychological counseling, and others are drop-in centers that offer everything from crash pads to free schools. All of them, however, can make referrals for medical help.

It's very important to call any service on the phone before dropping in. Clinics often have different hours for different types of medical care, and you may need an appointment in advance. The hours listed in this directory are not necessarily the hours for medical care—they are the hours when you can reach someone over the phone for information. Services that have no hours listed can usually be reached during the daytime.

When you call a clinic, it's a good idea to ask about their

fees. Many of the places on this list are free, but some charge for medical services.

It's also a good idea to ask if the clinic will treat someone your age. Most of the services listed here will not give you any hassle about age. However, some are cautious about following the state laws—especially when it comes to giving out birth control. If you find out the policy in advance, you can be prepared to lie about your age or sign any consent forms that are required.

If you live in a city that is not listed in this directory, there are several things you can do. You can find your local health department in the phone book, and a local hospital may also offer the kind of help you need. Check with the information operator to see if there is a Planned Parenthood chapter in your city. A hotline in a neighboring town may also be able to make referrals for your city.

If you can't find any health facilities in your area, there are some national services listed on p. 238. They will try to help you find what you're looking for.

ALABAMA

Clergy Consultation Service on Abortion
(205) 887-7182
Statewide referral service for pregnancy tests and abortions.

Birmingham

Freedom House
1207 15th St. S.
Birmingham, Alabama
(205) 323-2568
Free clinic offers birth control, pregnancy tests, VD treatment, general medical care, abortion referral, legal help, and general counseling. 1 P.M.–1 A.M. 7 days a week.

Crisis Center of Jefferson County
711 N. 18th St.
Birmingham, Alabama
(205) 323-7777
Hotline and counseling service; refers for birth control, pregnancy tests, VD tests, abortion, and legal help. 24 hours, 7 days a week.

Planned Parenthood—Birmingham Area
1714 11th Ave. S.
Birmingham, Alabama
(205) 933-8444
Offers birth control, pregnancy tests, VD tests, and abortion referral.

Huntsville

Huntsville Emergency Line
PO Box 92
Huntsville, Alabama
(205) 539-3424
Hotline and counseling service; refers

for birth control, pregnancy tests, VD tests, abortion, and legal help. 24 hours, 7 days a week.

Planned Parenthood Association of Madison County
304 Eustis Ave.
Huntsville, Alabama
(205) 534-0211
Offers birth control, pregnancy tests, VD tests, and abortion referral.

Mobile

Help Line
Mobile, Alabama
(205) 432-0711
Hotline refers for birth control, pregnancy tests, VD tests, abortion, and legal help. 4 P.M.–10 P.M. 7 days a week.

Montgomery

Help-a-Crisis Service
750 Washington Ave.
Montgomery, Alabama
(205) 265-9576
Hotline refers for birth control, pregnancy tests, VD tests, abortion, and legal help. 24 hours, 7 days a week.

Tuscaloosa

Planned Parenthood Association of Tuscaloosa
916 5th Ave. E.
Tuscaloosa, Alabama
(205) 758-9066
Offers birth control, pregnancy tests, VD tests, and abortion referral.

ALASKA

Anchorage

Open Door Clinic
513 E. 6th Ave.
Anchorage, Alaska
(907) 279-7561
Free clinic offers birth control, pregnancy tests, VD tests, general medical care, abortion referral, legal help, and general counseling. Makes referrals throughout the state. 24 hours, 7 days a week.

Family Planning
Greater Anchorage Area Health Department
630 Cordova
Anchorage, Alaska
(907) 279-2511
Public health clinic offers birth control and pregnancy tests.

ARIZONA

Clergy Consultation Service on Abortion
(602) 967-4234
Statewide referral service for pregnancy tests and abortions.

Mesa

Mesa Hotline
PO Box 74
Mesa, Arizona
(602) 969-5511
Hotline and counseling service; refers for birth control, pregnancy tests, VD tests, abortion, and legal help. 6 P.M.–midnight Mon.–Fri., 6 P.M.–2 A.M. Sat.–Sun.

Phoenix

Terros
502 W. Roosevelt
Phoenix, Arizona
(602) 257-8118
Free clinic and hotline; offers birth control, pregnancy tests, VD treatment, general medical care. Makes referrals for abortion and legal help. 24 hours, 7 days a week.

Planned Parenthood Association of Phoenix
1200 S. 5th Ave.
Phoenix, Arizona
(602) 257-1515
Offers birth control, pregnancy tests, VD tests, and abortion referral.

Community Information and Referral Service
1515 E. Osborn Rd.
Phoenix, Arizona
(602) 263-8856
Hotline refers for birth control, pregnancy tests, VD tests, abortion, and legal help. 8:30 A.M.–5 P.M. Mon.–Fri.

Tucson

Free Clinic of Tucson
256 S. Scott
Tucson, Arizona
(602) 622-8821
Free clinic offers birth control, pregnancy tests, VD treatment, general medical care, abortion referral, and general counseling. 6 P.M.–9 P.M. Tues. and Fri.

Planned Parenthood Center of Tucson
127 S. 5th Ave.
Tucson, Arizona
(602) 624-7477
Offers birth control, pregnancy tests, VD tests, and abortion referral.

Information and Referral
3833 E. 2nd St.
Tucson, Arizona
(602) 881-1794
Hotline refers for birth control, pregnancy tests, VD tests, abortion, and legal help. 9 A.M.–5 P.M. Mon.–Fri.

ARKANSAS

Little Rock

Switchboard
20th and Broadway
Little Rock, Arkansas
(501) 376-9141
Hotline refers for birth control, pregnancy tests, VD tests, abortion, and legal help. 5 P.M.–midnight Mon.–Thur., 5 P.M.–6 A.M. Fri.–Sun.

Contact
U.A.M.C. Box 225
4301 W. Markham
Little Rock, Arkansas
(501) 666-0234
Hotline refers for birth control, pregnancy tests, VD tests, abortion, and legal help. 24 hours, 7 days a week.

Hot Springs

Contact
Ouachita Regional Counseling
124 Rugg St.
Hot Springs, Arkansas
(501) 623-2515

Hotline refers for birth control, pregnancy tests, VD tests, and abortion.

CALIFORNIA

Alameda

Alameda Switchboard
PO Box 1185
Alameda, California
(415) 522-8363
Hotline refers for birth control, pregnancy tests, VD tests, abortion, and legal help. 4 P.M.–10 P.M. Mon.–Fri.

Anaheim

Free Clinic of Orange County
500-A N. Anaheim Blvd.
Anaheim, California
(714) 956-1900
Free clinic offers birth control, pregnancy tests, VD treatment, general medical care, abortion referral, legal help, and general counseling. 1 P.M.–10 P.M. Mon.–Thurs., 1 P.M.–5 P.M. Fri.

Berkeley

Berkeley Community Clinic
2339 Durant Ave.
Berkeley, California
(415) 548-2570
Free clinic offers VD tests and general medical care. Makes referrals for pregnancy tests, birth control, and abortion. Afternoons Mon.–Fri.

Berkeley Women's Health Collective
2214 Grove St.
Berkeley, California
(415) 843-6194
Women's center offers counseling and referral for birth control and abortion.

Fresno

Planned Parenthood of Fresno
404 W. McKinley
Fresno, California
(209) 486-2411
Offers birth control, pregnancy tests, VD tests, and abortion referral. Special teen clinics.

Hayward

Planned Parenthood of Hayward
1252 B St.
Hayward, California
(415) 538-6330
Offers birth control, pregnancy tests, VD tests, and abortion referral. Special teen clinics.

Hollywood

Hollywood-Sunset Free Clinic
3324 Sunset Blvd.
Hollywood, California
(213) 660-2400
Free clinic offers birth control, pregnancy tests, VD treatment, general medical care, abortion referral, and legal help. 10 A.M.–10 P.M. Mon.–Fri.

Los Angeles

Los Angeles Free Clinic
115 N. Fairfax
Los Angeles, California
(213) 938-9141
Free clinic offers birth control, pregnancy tests, VD treatment, general medical care, abortion referral,

legal help, and general counseling. 1 P.M.–10 P.M. Mon.–Fri.

Northeast Youth Clinic
2032 Marengo St.
Los Angeles, California
(213) 225-5971
(213) 225-0679 after 5 P.M.
Free clinic offers birth control, pregnancy tests, VD treatment, general medical care, abortion referral, and general counseling. 4:30–8:30 P.M. Mon., Wed., Thurs., Fri.

Imperial Heights Youth Clinic
10616 S. Western Ave.
Los Angeles, California
(213) 757-9171
Free clinic offers birth control, pregnancy tests, VD treatment, general medical care, and abortion referral. 3:30—8:30 P.M. Mon.—Fri.

Planned Parenthood–World Population
3100 W. 8th St.
Los Angeles, California
(213) 380-9300
Offers birth control, pregnancy tests, VD tests, and abortion referral.

Feminist Women's Health Center
746 Crenshaw Blvd.
Los Angeles, California
(213) 936-7466
Women's clinic offers birth control, pregnancy tests, VD tests, gynecological care, and abortion. 24 hours, 7 days a week.

The Women's Clinic
6423 Wilshire Blvd.
Suite 105
Los Angeles, California
(213) 655-5410
Women's clinic offers birth control, pregnancy tests, VD treatment, gynecological care, and abortion. Noon–9 P.M. Mon.–Fri.

Legal Switchboard
Los Angeles, California
(213) 6-MOTHER
Hotline offers legal information and help.

Crenshaw Hotline
4436 W. 62nd St.
Los Angeles, California
(213) 299-6666
Hotline refers for birth control, pregnancy tests, VD tests, and abortion. 6 P.M.–10 P.M. Tues.–Sat.

Westchester Hotline
8015 S. Sepulveda Blvd.
Los Angeles, California
(213) 645-3333
Hotline refers for birth control, pregnancy tests, VD tests, and abortion. 24 hours, 7 days a week.

Mountain View

Planned Parenthood
251 Moffett Blvd.
Mountain View, California
(415) 961-6839
Referral service for birth control, pregnancy tests, VD tests, and abortion. 11 A.M.—5 P.M. Mon.—Fri.

Oakland

Planned Parenthood–World Population of Alameda–San Francisco
476 W. MacArthur Blvd.
Oakland, California
(415) 654-7987
Offers birth control, pregnancy tests,

VD tests, and abortion referral. Special teen clinics.

East Oakland Planned Parenthood Center
9810 E. 14th St.
East Oakland, California
(415) 562-1103
Offers birth control, pregnancy tests, VD tests, and abortion referral. Special teen clinics.

Orange

Planned Parenthood Association of Orange County
704 N. Glassell
Orange, California
(714) 639-3023
Offers birth control, pregnancy tests, VD tests, and abortion referral.

Pacific Grove

Planned Parenthood of Monterey County, Inc.
216 17th St.
Pacific Grove, California
(408) 373-1691
Offers birth control, pregnancy tests, abortion referral.

Pasadena

Pasadena Planned Parenthood Committee, Inc.
1045 N. Lake Ave.
Pasadena, California
(213) 798-0706
Offers birth control, pregnancy tests, VD tests, and abortion referral.

Pleasanton

Planned Parenthood of Pleasanton
4361 Railroad Ave.
Pleasanton, California
(415) 462-1950
Offers birth control and abortion referral.

Richmond

Contra Costa Planned Parenthood, Richmond Center
255 Civic Center St.
Richmond, California
(415) 233-1900
Offers birth control, pregnancy tests, and abortion referral.

Sacramento

Aquarian Effort Free Clinic
1239 Q St.
Sacramento, California
(916) 444-6294
Free clinic and hotline offers birth control, pregnancy tests, VD treatment, general medical care, abortion referral, and legal help. 24 hours, 7 days a week.

Planned Parenthood Association of Sacramento
1507 21st St., Suite 100
Sacramento, California
(916) 446-5034
Offers birth control, pregnancy tests, and abortion referral.

San Diego

Beach Area Free Clinic
3705 Mission Blvd.
San Diego, California
(714) 488-0644
Free clinic offers birth control, pregnancy tests, VD treatment, general medical care, and abortion referral. 1 P.M.–10 P.M. Mon.–Sat.

Planned Parenthood Association of San Diego County
1172 Morena Blvd.
San Diego, California
(714) 276-9740
Offers birth control, pregnancy tests, and abortion referral. Special teen clinics.

San Francisco

San Francisco Sex Information
340 Jones St.
San Francisco, California
(415) 665-7300
Hotline and counseling service, refers for birth control, pregnancy tests, VD tests, and abortion. 3 P.M.–9 P.M. Mon.–Fri.

Planned Parenthood of San Francisco
2340 Clay St.
San Francisco, California
(415) 922-1720
Offers birth control, pregnancy tests, VD tests, and abortion referral. Special teen clinics.

District Health Center #1
3850 17th at Noe
San Francisco, California
(415) 558-3905
Public health clinic offers birth control, pregnancy tests, VD tests, and abortion referral.

District Health Center #2
1301 Pierce
San Francisco, California
(415) 558-3256
Public health clinic offers birth control, pregnancy tests, VD tests, and abortion referral.

District Health Center #3
1525 Silver Ave.
San Francisco, California
(415) 468-3664
Public health clinic offers birth control, pregnancy tests, VD tests, and abortion referral.

District Health Center #4
1490 Mason
San Francisco, California
(415) 558-2011
Public health clinic offers birth control, pregnancy tests, VD tests, and abortion referral.

District Health Center #5
1351 24th Ave.
San Francisco, California
(415) 558-3246
Public health clinic offers birth control, pregnancy tests, VD tests, and abortion referral.

San Francisco City Clinic
250 4th St.
San Francisco, California
(415) 558-3804
Public health clinic offers VD tests and treatment.

Haight-Ashbury Free Medical Clinic
558 Clayton
San Francisco, California
(415) 431-1714
Free clinic offers birth control, pregnancy tests, VD treatment, general medical care, and abortion referral. 9 A.M.–10 P.M. Mon.–Fri.

Bay Area Venereal Disease Association
(415) 668-7777
Hotline refers for VD tests and treatment throughout the San Francisco Greater Bay Area.

San Jose

Free Youth Clinic
1989 McKee Rd.
San Jose, California
(408) 251-2760
Free clinic offers birth control, pregnancy tests, VD treatment, general medical care, and abortion referral. 8 A.M.–5 P.M. Mon.–Fri.

Planned Parenthood Association of Santa Clara County
28 N. 16th St.
San Jose, California
(408) 294-3032
Offers birth control, pregnancy tests, and abortion referral. Special teen clinics.

San Mateo

Planned Parenthood of San Mateo County
373 S. Claremont
San Mateo, California
(415) 348-2424
Offers birth control, pregnancy tests, and abortion referral. Special teen clinics.

San Rafael

Planned Parenthood Association of Marin County
710 C St., Suite 9
San Rafael, California
(415) 454-0471
Offers birth control, pregnancy tests, VD tests, and abortion referral. Special teen clinics.

Santa Barbara

Planned Parenthood of Santa Barbara County
322 Palm Ave.
Santa Barbara, California
(805) 963-4417
Offers birth control, pregnancy tests, and abortion referral.

Santa Cruz

Planned Parenthood of Santa Cruz County
PO Box 1196
Santa Cruz, California
(408) 426-5550
Referral service for birth control, pregnancy tests, VD tests, and abortion.

Santa Monica

EX-HELPS
PO Box 3701
Santa Monica, California
(213) 394-3577
Hotline refers for birth control, pregnancy tests, VD tests, abortion, and legal help.

Stockton

Planned Parenthood of Joaquin County
116 W. Willow
Stockton, California
(209) 464-5809
Offers birth control, pregnancy tests, and abortion referral.

Walnut Creek

Planned Parenthood of Contra Costa County, Walnut Creek Center
1291 Oakland Blvd.
Walnut Creek, California
(415) 935-3010

Offers birth control, pregnancy tests, and abortion referral.

Woodland

Yolo County Health and Family Planning Association, Inc.
327 College St., Suite 102
Woodland, California
(916) 666-0707
Offers birth control, pregnancy tests, and abortion referral.

COLORADO

Clergy Consultation Service on Abortion
(303) 757-4442
Statewide referral service for pregnancy tests and abortion.

Boulder

People's Clinic
999 Alpine
Boulder, Colorado
(303) 449-6050
Free clinic offers birth control, pregnancy tests, VD treatment, general medical care, and abortion referral. 9 A.M.–5 P.M. Mon–Fri.

Planned Parenthood of Boulder
3450 Broadway
Boulder, Colorado
(303) 447-1040
Offers birth control, pregnancy tests, and abortion referral.

Colorado Springs

Youth Information Line
27 E. Vermijo
Colorado Springs, Colorado
(303) 471-5979
Hotline refers for birth control, pregnancy tests, VD tests, abortion, and legal help. 9 A.M.–5 P.M. Mon.–Fri.

Planned Parenthood of Colorado Springs
501 N. Foote
Colorado Springs, Colorado
(303) 634-3771
Offers birth control, pregnancy tests, and abortion referral. Special teen clinics.

Denver

Eastside Neighborhood Health Center
29th and Welton
Denver, Colorado
(303) 224-4661
Public health clinic offers birth control, pregnancy tests, VD treatment, general medical care, and abortion referral.

Westside Neighborhood Health Center
990 Federal Blvd.
Denver, Colorado
(303) 292-9690
Public health clinic offers birth control, pregnancy tests, VD treatment, general medical care, and abortion referral.

Hip Help and Denver Free Clinic
1304 Elati
Denver, Colorado
(303) 222-3344
Free clinic offers birth control, pregnancy tests, VD treatment, and abortion referral. 24 hours, 7 days a week.

Rocky Mountain Planned Parenthood

2030 E. 20th Ave.
Denver, Colorado
(303) 388-4215
Offers birth control, pregnancy tests, and abortion referral.

Connection
1777 Clarkson
Denver, Colorado
(303) 892-1812
Hotline refers for birth control, pregnancy tests, VD tests, abortion, and legal help. 9 A.M.–9 P.M. Mon.–Fri.

Greeley

Planned Parenthood of Greeley
1555 17th Ave.
Greeley, Colorado
(303) 353-0540
Offers birth control, pregnancy tests, and abortion referral.

Pueblo

Planned Parenthood of Pueblo
151 Central Main
Pueblo, Colorado
(303) 545-0246
Offers birth control, pregnancy tests, and abortion referral. Special teen clinics.

CONNECTICUT

Clergy Consultation Service on Abortion
(203) 624-8646
Statewide referral service for pregnancy tests and abortions.

Bridgeport

Bridgeport Planned Parenthood
1067 Park Ave.
Bridgeport, Connecticut
(203) 366-0664
Offers birth control, pregnancy tests, VD tests, and abortion referral.

Danbury

Danbury Planned Parenthood
240 Main St.
Danbury, Connecticut
(203) 743-2446
Referral service makes arrangements for birth control and pregnancy tests. 10 A.M.–2 P.M. Mon.–Fri.

Darien

Centre Stone
1081 Post Rd.
Darien, Connecticut
(203) 655-1485
Hotline and counseling service, refers for birth control, pregnancy tests, VD tests, abortion, and legal help. Noon–midnight Sun.–Fri., all night Sat.

Greenwich

Greenwich Hotline
116 W. Putnam St.
Greenwich, Connecticut
(203) 661-4357
Hotline refers for birth control, pregnancy tests, VD tests, abortion, and legal help. 4 P.M.–9 P.M. Sun.–Thurs., 4 P.M.–2 A.M. Fri.–Sat.

Hartford

Roots
109 Allyn St.
Hartford, Connecticut

(203) 525-1131
Hotline refers for birth control, pregnancy tests, VD tests, abortion, and legal help. 24 hours, 7 days a week.

Hartford Planned Parenthood
293 Farmington Ave.
Hartford, Connecticut
(203) 522-6201
Offers birth control, pregnancy tests, abortion referral. Special teen clinics.

Meriden

Helpline
22 Liberty St.
Meriden, Connecticut
(203 238-2266
Hotline refers for birth control, pregnancy tests, VD tests, abortion, and legal help. 24 hours, 7 days a week.

Meriden/Wallingford Planned Parenthood
PO Box 2119
Meriden, Connecticut
(203) 235-3231
Referral service for birth control, pregnancy tests, and abortion.

Middletown

Touch
115 College St.
Middletown, Connecticut
(203) 344-0315
Hotline refers for birth control, pregnancy tests, VD tests, abortion, and legal help. 24 hours, 7 days a week.

Middlesex Planned Parenthood
60 Crescent St.
Middletown, Connecticut
(203) 347-5255
Offers birth control, pregnancy tests, and abortion referral.

New Britain

New Britain Planned Parenthood
PO Box 292
New Britain, Connecticut
(203) 225-9811
Referral service for birth control, pregnancy tests, and abortion.

New Haven

Number Nine
266 State St.
New Haven, Connecticut
(203) 787-2127
Hotline refers for birth control, pregnancy tests, VD tests, abortion, and legal help. 6 P.M.–midnight 7 days a week.

Planned Parenthood League of Connecticut
406 Orange St.
New Haven, Connecticut
(203) 865-0595
Offers birth control, pregnancy tests, and abortion referral.

Information and Referral Service
1 State St.
New Haven, Connecticut
(203) 624-3136
Hotline refers for birth control, pregnancy tests, VD tests, abortion, and legal help. 9 A.M.–5 P.M. Mon.–Fri.

New London

Southeastern Planned Parenthood

160 Shaw St.
New London, Connecticut
(203) 443-5820
Offers birth control, pregnancy tests, and abortion referral. 8:30–3:30 Mon.–Fri.

Norwich

Southeastern Planned Parenthood
325 Washington St.
Norwich, Connecticut
(203) 887-8962
Offers birth control, pregnancy tests, and abortion referral. 8:30–3:30 Mon.–Fri.

Stamford

Southern Fairfield Planned Parenthood
259 Main St.
Stamford, Connecticut
(203) 327-2722
Offers birth control, pregnancy tests, and abortion referral.

Waterbury

Waterbury Planned Parenthood
59 Cooke St.
Waterbury, Connecticut
(203) 757-1955
Offers birth control, pregnancy tests, and abortion referral.

Willimantic

Northeastern Chapter, Planned Parenthood
132 Valley St.
Willimantic, Connecticut
(203) 423-1500
Offers birth control, pregnancy tests, and abortion referral.

DELAWARE

Newark

Dial
Newark, Delaware
(302) 738-5555
Hotline refers for birth control, pregnancy tests, VD tests, abortion, and legal help. 8 A.M.–2 A.M. Mon.–Fri.

Wilmington

Delaware League for Planned Parenthood
825 Washington St.
Wilmington, Delaware
(302) 655-7293
Offers birth control, pregnancy tests, and abortion referral.

DISTRICT OF COLUMBIA

Also check listings under Maryland and Virginia for other services in the D.C. area.

Washington Free Clinic
1556 Wisconsin Ave. NW
Washington, D.C.
(202) 965-5476
Free clinic offers birth control, pregnancy tests, VD tests, general medical care, abortion referral and legal help. 6:30 P.M.–10 P.M.

The Gate Health Clinic
3336 M St. NW
Washington, D.C.
(202) 337-4283
Free clinic offers birth control, pregnancy tests, VD tests, general medical care, and abortion referral.

Planned Parenthood of Metropolitan Washington, D.C.
1109 M St., NW
Washington, D.C.
(202) 387-8787
Offers birth control, pregnancy tests, and abortion referral. Special teen clinics.

Pregnancy Testing, Counseling and Abortion Referral Service
1112 M St. NW
Washington, D.C.
(202) 462-1358
Offers pregnancy tests and abortion referral.

Northwest Central Clinic
1325 Upshire St. NW
Washington, D.C.
(202) 629-7578
Public health clinic offers birth control, pregnancy tests, VD treatment, and general medical care.

Georgetown Legal Interns
600 New Jersey Ave. NW
Washington, D.C.
(202) 624-8380
Counseling service, offers legal information and help.

George Washington University Legal Aid Bureau
714 21st St. NW
Washington, D.C.
(202) 676-7163
Counseling service, offers legal information and help.

Public Health Department
VD Hotline
Washington, D.C.
(202) VD 2-7000
Referral service for VD tests and treatment.

Human Resources Information and Referral Service
919 12th St. NW
Washington, D.C.
(202) 629-3776
Health department referral service for birth control, pregnancy tests, VD tests, and abortion.

FLORIDA

Clergy Consultation Service on Abortion
(305) 372-5883
Statewide referral service for pregnancy tests and abortions.

Gainesville

Corner Drugstore
1128 SW 1st Ave.
Gainesville, Florida
(904) 378-1588
Free clinic and hotline, offers birth control, pregnancy tests, VD treatment, general medical care, abortion referral, and general counseling. 24 hours, 7 days a week.

Jacksonville

Planned Parenthood of Northeast Florida
Universal Marion Building, Suite 1010
Jacksonville, Florida
(904) 354-7796
Offers birth control, pregnancy tests, and abortion referral. Special teen clinics.

Miami

Women's Medical Center and Family Planning Service
7821 Coral Way
Miami, Florida
(305) 444-8213
Free clinic offers birth control, pregnancy tests, VD treatment, general medical care, and abortion referral.

Switchboard of Miami
2175 SW 26th St.
Miami, Florida
(305) 634-1511
Hotline refers for birth control, pregnancy tests, VD tests, abortion, and legal help. 24 hours, 7 days a week.

Orlando

Teenage Hotline
610 Mariposa
Orlando, Florida
(305) 644-2027
Hotline refers for birth control, pregnancy tests, VD tests, abortion, and legal help. 4 P.M.–midnight 7 days a week.

We Care
610 Mariposa
Orlando, Florida
(305) 241-3329
Hotline refers for birth control, pregnancy tests, VD tests, abortion, and legal help. 24 hours, 7 days a week.

Planned Parenthood of Central Florida
106 W. Central Blvd.
Orlando, Florida
(305) 425-5514
Referral service for birth control, pregnancy tests, VD tests, and abortion.

St. Petersburg

St. Petersburg Hotline
4635 17th Ave. S.
St. Petersburg, Florida
(813) 896-7101
Hotline and counseling service, refers for birth control, pregnancy tests, VD tests, abortion, and legal help. 9 A.M.–midnight.

Sarasota

Planned Parenthood Association of Sarasota
1224 S. Tamiami Trail
Sarasota, Florida
(813) 959-2439
Offers birth control, pregnancy tests, and abortion referral.

Tallahassee

Project 613
733 W. Pensacola
Tallahassee, Florida
(904) 599-9596
Hotline refers for birth control, pregnancy tests, VD tests, abortion, and legal help. 24 hours, 7 days a week.

Tampa

The Door

1718 W. Casf St.
Tampa, Florida
(813) 251-1001
Hotline refers for birth control, pregnancy tests, VD tests, abortion, and legal help. 24 hours, 7 days a week.

West Palm Beach

Planned Parenthood–Palm Beach Area
120 South Olive Ave.
West Palm Beach, Florida
(305) 655-7984
Offers birth control, pregnancy tests, abortion referral.

GEORGIA

Atlanta

Community Crisis Center
1013 Peachtree St. NE
Atlanta, Georgia
(404) 892-1358
Free clinic and hotline offers birth control, pregnancy tests, VD treatment, general medical care, abortion referral, and general counseling. 24 hours, 7 days a week.

Northeast Health Center and Family Planning Clinic
626 Parkway Drive, NE
Atlanta, Georgia
(404) 876-0305
Free clinic offers birth control, pregnancy tests, VD treatment, and general medical care. 9 A.M.–5 P.M. Mon.–Fri.

Planned Parenthood Association of the Atlanta Area
118 Marietta St.
Atlanta, Georgia
(404) 688-9300
Offers birth control, pregnancy tests, and abortion referral. 9 A.M.–8 P.M. Mon.–Fri., 9 A.M.–4 P.M. Sat.

Public Health Department
Atlanta, Georgia
(404) 572-2201
Public health department referral service for pregnancy tests and VD tests.

Augusta

Planned Parenthood of East Central Georgia
1862 Central Ave.
Augusta, Georgia
(404) 736-1161
Offers birth control, pregnancy tests, and abortion referral.

Savannah

Helpline
1512 Bull St.
Savannah, Georgia
(912) 233-0146
Hotline and counseling service, refers for birth control, pregnancy tests, VD tests, abortion, and legal help. 8 A.M.–10 P.M. Mon.–Fri.

HAWAII

Honolulu

Hawaii Planned Parenthood Center
200 North Vineyard Blvd., Suite 501
Honolulu, Oahu

(808) 537-5557
Offers birth control, pregnancy tests, and abortion referral.

Information and Referral Service
200 North Vineyard Blvd., Suite 603
Honolulu, Oahu
(808) 521-4566
Hotline refers for birth control, pregnancy tests, VD tests, abortion, and legal help. 24 hours, 7 days a week.

Hilo

Planned Parenthood of Hilo
46 Keawe St.
Hilo, Hawaii
(808) 935-1320
Referral service for birth control, pregnancy tests, and abortion.

Lihue

Planned Parenthood of Kauai
2786 Wehe Road
Lihue, Kauai
(808) 245-6473
Referral service for birth control, pregnancy tests, VD tests, and abortion.

Wailuku

Hawaii Planned Parenthood of Maui
1995 Main St., Suite 3
Wailuku, Maui
Offers birth control, pregnancy tests, VD tests, and abortion referral.

IDAHO

Boise

Youth Service Bureau
807 Franklin
Boise, Idaho
(208) 354-9337
Referral service for birth control, pregnancy tests, VD tests, abortion, and legal help. 8 A.M.–5 P.M. Mon.–Fri.

Hotline of Boise
PO Box 235
Boise, Idaho
(208) 376-2555
Hotline refers for birth control, pregnancy tests, VD tests, abortion, and legal help. 7 P.M.–3 A.M. 7 days a week.

Planned Parenthood Association of Idaho
PO Box 264
Boise, Idaho
(208) 345-0760
Referral service for birth control, pregnancy tests, and VD tests.

Caldwell

Hotline
PO Box 1104
Caldwell, Idaho
(208) 466-3511
Hotline refers for birth control, pregnancy tests, VD tests, abortion, and legal help. 7 P.M.–11 P.M. 7 days a week.

ILLINOIS

Clergy Consultation Service on Abortion
(312) 667-6015
Statewide referral service for pregnancy tests and abortions.

Bloomington

Planned Parenthood of McLean County
210 E. Washington
Bloomington, Illinois
(309) 829-3028
Offers birth control, pregnancy tests, VD tests, and abortion referral.

Champaign

Planned Parenthood Association of Champaign County
505 S. 5th St.
Champaign, Illinois
(217) 359-8022
Offers birth control, pregnancy tests, VD tests, and abortion referral. Special teen clinics.

Hotline for Youth
1206 S. Randolph
Champaign, Illinois
(217) 359-8020
Hotline refers for birth control, pregnancy tests, VD tests, abortion, and legal help.

Francis Nelson Free Clinic
1306 Carver
Champaign, Illinois
(217) 356-1558
Free clinic offers birth control, pregnancy tests, VD treatment, and general medical care. 9 A.M.–5 P.M. Mon.–Fri.

Chicago

Metro-Help
2210 N. Halsted
Chicago, Illinois
(312) 929-5150
Hotline refers for birth control, pregnancy tests, VD tests, abortion, and legal help. 24 hours, 7 days a week.

Planned Parenthood Association–Chicago Area
185 N. Wabash Ave.
Chicago, Illinois
(312) 726-5134
Offers birth control, pregnancy tests, VD tests, and abortion referral. Special teen clinics.

Fritzi Engelstein Free People's Clinic
2747 N. Wilton St.
Chicago, Illinois
(312) 348-8578
Free clinic offers birth control, pregnancy tests, and general medical care. 6 P.M.–9 P.M. Tues. and Wed.

Young Patriots Clinic
4403 Sheridan
Chicago, Illinois
(312) 334-8957
Free clinic offers birth control, pregnancy tests, VD tests, and general medical care. 7:30 P.M.–10 P.M. Mon. and Thurs.

Chicago Board of Health
Municipal Social Hygiene Clinic
27 E. 26th St.
Chicago, Illinois
(312) 842-0222
Public health department makes referrals for VD tests and treatment.

Northwestern Legal Clinic
360 E. Superior
Chicago, Illinois
(312) 649-8576
Hotline offers legal information and help.

Chicago Volunteer Legal Services
19 S. LaSalle

Chicago, Illinois
(312) 332-1624
Legal agency offers information and help.

Decatur

Planned Parenthood of Decatur
919 N. Water St.
Decatur, Illinois
(217) 429-9211
Offers birth control, pregnancy tests, VD tests, and abortion referral.

Freeport

People's Free Medical Clinic
530 W. Main St.
Freeport, Illinois
(815) 232-8403
Free clinic offers birth control, pregnancy tests, VD treatment, general medical care, and abortion referral. 9 A.M.–5 P.M. Mon.–Fri.

Joliet

Lemonade
216 E. Cass St.
Joliet, Illinois
(815) 727-4615
Hotline refers for birth control, pregnancy tests, VD tests, abortion, and legal help.

Oak Park

Oak Park Hotline
255 Augusta
Oak Park, Illinois
(312) 848-2555
Hotline refers for birth control, pregnancy tests, VD tests, abortion, and legal help. 6 P.M.–6 A.M. 7 days a week.

Peoria

Planned Parenthood Association of the Peoria Area
509 W. High St.
Peoria, Illinois
(309) 673-6911
Offers birth control, pregnancy tests, and abortion referral.

Rockford

Contact Rockford
Box 2179
Rockford, Illinois
(815) 877-4044
Hotline refers for birth control, pregnancy tests, VD tests, and abortion. 24 hours, 7 days a week.

INDIANA

Clergy Consultation Service on Abortion
(219) 422-2288
Statewide referral service for pregnancy tests and abortions.

Bloomington

Planned Parenthood Association of Monroe County
406 S. College Ave.
Bloomington, Indiana
(812) 336-0219
Offers birth control, pregnancy tests, VD tests, and abortion referral.

Evansville

Youth Service Bureau
203 NW 5th St.
Evansville, Indiana

(812) 425-4355
Referral service for birth control, pregnancy tests, VD tests, abortion, and legal help.

Planned Parenthood of Evansville
1610 S. Weinbach
Evansville, Indiana
(812) 479-1466
Offers birth control and abortion referral.

Fort Wayne

Switchboard
1012 Broadway
Fort Wayne, Indiana
(219) 742-7333
Hotline refers for birth control, pregnancy tests, VD tests, abortion, and legal help. 24 hours, 7 days a week.

Gary

Planned Parenthood of Northwestern Indiana
740 Washington St.
Gary, Indiana
(219) 883-0411
Offers birth control, pregnancy tests, VD tests, and abortion referral.

Indianapolis

Dawn Line
6105 Guilford
Indianapolis, Indiana
(317) 257-3296
Hotline refers for birth control, pregnancy tests, VD tests, abortion, and legal help. 3 P.M.–3 A.M. 7 days a week.

Planned Parenthood Association of Indianapolis
615 N. Alabama St., Room 332
Indianapolis, Indiana
(317) 634-8019
Offers birth control, pregnancy tests, abortion referral.

Lafayette

Planned Parenthood Association of Tippecanoe County
602 Columbia St.
Lafayette, Indiana
(317) 742-5886
Referral service for birth control, pregnancy tests, VD tests, and abortion.

Muncie

Planned Parenthood of Delaware County
261 Johnston Building
Muncie, Indiana
(317) 282-8011
Offers birth control, pregnancy tests, and abortion referral.

South Bend

Hotline
1011 E. Madison St.
South Bend, Indiana
(219) 282-2323
Hotline refers for birth control, pregnancy tests, VD tests, abortion, and legal help.

Planned Parenthood of North Central Indiana
201 S. Chapin
South Bend, Indiana
(219) 289-7027
Offers birth control, pregnancy tests, and abortion referral.

Terre Haute

Planned Parenthood of Vigo County
1024 S. 6th St.
Terre Haute, Indiana
(812) 232-4852
Offers birth control, pregnancy tests, and abortion referral.

IOWA

Clergy Consultation Service on Abortion
(515) 282-1738
Statewide referral service for pregnancy tests and abortions.

Burlington

Planned Parenthood of Des Moines County
521 N. 5th St.
Burlington, Iowa
(319) 753-2281
Offers birth control, pregnancy tests, VD tests, and abortion referral.

Des Moines

Youth Line
Lutheran Hospital
E. 7th and University
Des Moines, Iowa
(515) 265-7333
Hotline and counseling service, refers for birth control, pregnancy tests, VD tests, abortion, and legal help. 9 A.M.–midnight 7 days a week.

Planned Parenthood of Iowa
851 19th St.
Des Moines, Iowa
(515) 280-7000
Offers birth control, pregnancy tests, and abortion referral.

Iowa City

Iowa City Free Medical Clinic
120 N. Dubuque
Iowa City, Iowa
(319) 337-4459
Free clinic offers birth control, pregnancy tests, VD treatment, general medical care, and abortion referral. Noon–5 P.M. Mon.–Fri.

Iowa City Crisis Intervention Center
608 S. Dubuque
Iowa City, Iowa
(319) 351-0140
Hotline and counseling service, refers for birth control, pregnancy tests, VD tests, abortion, and legal help. 11 A.M.–2 A.M. 7 days a week.

Keokuk

Planned Parenthood of Southeast Iowa
927 Exchange St.
Keokuk, Iowa
(319) 524-2759
Offers birth control, pregnancy tests, VD tests, and abortion referral.

Mt. Pleasant

Planned Parenthood of Henry County
Human Services, Mental Health Institute
Mt. Pleasant, Iowa
(319) 385-4310
Offers birth control, pregnancy tests, VD tests, and abortion referral.

Sioux City

Sioux City Hotline
PO Box 2711
Sioux City, Iowa
(712) 276-0821
Hotline refers for birth control, pregnancy tests, VD tests, abortion, and legal help. 6 P.M.–1 A.M. 7 days a week.

Planned Parenthood Committee of Sioux City
2825 Douglas St.
Sioux City, Iowa
(712) 258-4019
Offers birth control, pregnancy tests, and abortion referral.

Washington

Planned Parenthood of Washington County
Washington County Hospital
Washington, Iowa
(319) 653-3525
Offers birth control, pregnancy tests, VD tests, and problem-pregnancy counseling.

Waterloo

Crisis Line
YMCA Building
Waterloo, Iowa
(319) 234-6603
Hotline refers for birth control, pregnancy tests, VD tests, abortion, and legal help. 24 hours, 7 days a week.

Planned Parenthood of Northeast Iowa
604 Mulberry
Waterloo, Iowa
(319) 235-6243
Referral service for birth control, pregnancy tests, VD tests, and abortion.

KANSAS

Clergy Consultation Service on Abortion
(913) 539-3011
Statewide referral service for pregnancy tests and abortions.

Hutchinson

Hotline
14 East 2nd St.
Hutchinson, Kansas
(316) 663-2701
Hotline refers for birth control, pregnancy tests, VD tests, abortion, and legal help. 24 hours, 7 days a week.

Kansas City

Hotline
5424 State Ave.
Kansas City, Kansas
(913) 287-1300
Hotline refers for birth control, pregnancy tests, VD tests, abortion, and legal help. 6 P.M.–midnight 7 days a week.

Planned Parenthood Association of Western Missouri/Kansas
4950 Cherry St.
Kansas City, Missouri
(816) 931-4121
Offers birth control, pregnancy tests, and abortion referral.

Lawrence

Headquarters

1632 Kentucky
Lawrence, Kansas
(913) 841-2345
Hotline and counseling service, refers for birth control, pregnancy tests, VD tests, and abortion. 24 hours, 7 days a week.

Topeka

Can Help
PO Box 4253
Topeka, Kansas
(913) 235-3434
Hotline refers for birth control, pregnancy tests, VD tests, and abortion. 24 hours, 7 days a week.

Wichita

Wichita Red Cross Hotline
321 N. Topeka
Wichita, Kansas
(316) 265-8577
Hotline refers for birth control, pregnancy tests, VD tests, and abortion.

KENTUCKY

Berea

The Mountain Maternal Health League
211 Municipal Building
Berea, Kentucky
(606) 986-4677
Planned Parenthood, offers birth control, pregnancy tests, and abortion referral.

Lexington

Crisis Intervention Service
201 Mechanic St.
Lexington, Kentucky
(606) 254-3844
Hotline and counseling service, refers for birth control, pregnancy tests, VD tests, and abortion. 24 hours, 7 days a week.

Lexington Planned Parenthood Center
331 W. 2nd St.
Lexington, Kentucky
(606) 255-4913
Offers birth control, pregnancy tests, and abortion referral.

Louisville

Hair
522 E. Gray St.
Louisville, Kentucky
(502) 589-4470
Hotline refers for birth control, pregnancy tests, VD tests, abortion, and legal help. 24 hours, 7 days a week.

Planned Parenthood Center
843-845 Barret Ave.
Louisville, Kentucky
(502) 584-2471
Offers birth control, pregnancy tests, and abortion referral.

LOUISIANA

Clergy Consultation Service on Abortion
(504) 897-6980

Baton Rouge

The Phone
Student Health Service
Louisiana State University
Baton Rouge, Louisiana
(504) 388-8222

Hotline refers for birth control, pregnancy tests, VD tests, abortion, and legal help.

New Orleans

H.E.A.D. Clinic
(Health Emergency Aid Dispensary)
1130 N. Rampart
New Orleans, Louisiana
(504) 524-1446
Free clinic offers birth control, pregnancy tests, VD tests, general medical care, and abortion referral. 6 P.M.–9 P.M. Mon., Tues., Thurs., Fri.

N.O.S.E.
(New Orleans Switchboard Exchange)
1212 Royal St.
New Orleans, Louisiana
(504) 524-9314
Hotline and counseling service, refers for birth control, pregnancy tests, VD tests, abortion, and legal help. 24 hours, 7 days a week.

MAINE

Clergy Consultation Service on Abortion
(207) 773-3866
Statewide referral service for pregnancy tests and abortions.

Bangor

Dial Help
43 Illinois Ave.
Bangor, Maine
(207) 947-6143 local callers
(800) 432-7810 statewide callers
Hotline and counseling service, refers for birth control, pregnancy tests, VD tests, abortion, and legal help. 24 hours, 7 days a week.

Lewistown

Rap Place
145 Park St.
Lewistown, Maine
(207) 784-1564
Hotline refers for birth control, pregnancy tests, VD tests, abortion, and legal help. 24 hours, 7 days a week.

Portland

Health Department
City Hall
389 Congress St.
Portland, Maine
(207) 775-5451
Public health department clinic for VD tests and treatment. Makes referrals for birth control, pregnancy tests, and abortions. 8 A.M.–5 P.M. Mon.–Fri.

Family Planning Clinic
681 Congress St.
Portland, Maine
(207) 774-3996
Offers birth control. Makes referrals for pregnancy tests and abortions. 8 A.M.–5 P.M. Mon.–Fri.

MARYLAND

Annapolis

Public Health Department
3 Broad Creek Parkway
Annapolis, Maryland
(301) 267-8151
Makes referrals for birth control, pregnancy tests, VD tests, general medical care, and abortion.

Baltimore

Planned Parenthood Association of Maryland
517 N. Charles St.
Baltimore, Maryland
(301) 752-0131
Offers birth control and abortion referral.

Pregnancy Testing and Counseling Service
809 Cathedral St.
Baltimore, Maryland
(301) 752-2161
Offers pregnancy tests and abortion referral.

People's Free Medical Clinic
3028 Greenmount Ave.
Baltimore, Maryland
(301) 467-6040
Free clinic for Waverly residents. Offers birth control, pregnancy tests, VD tests, and general medical care. Noon–10 P.M. Mon.–Thurs.

Hotline for Youth
PO Box 5959
Baltimore, Maryland
(301) 653-2000
Hotline refers for birth control, pregnancy tests, VD tests, abortion, and legal help. 7 P.M.–2 A.M. 7 days a week.

Bethesda

Listening Post
10300 W. Lake Drive
Bethesda, Maryland
(301) 469-9212
Hotline and counseling service, refers for birth control, pregnancy tests, VD tests, abortion, and legal help. 3 P.M.–10 P.M. Mon–Fri.

Catonsville

Lighthouse
616 S. Rolling Rd.
Catonsville, Maryland
(301) 788-5483
Hotline and counseling service, refers for birth control, pregnancy tests, VD tests, abortion, and legal help. Noon–midnight 7 days a week.

Frederick

Frederick County Hotline
500 W. Patrick St.
Frederick, Maryland
(301) 662-9444
Hotline and counseling service, refers for birth control, pregnancy tests, VD tests, abortion, and legal help. 6 P.M.–midnight 7 days a week.

Hagerstown

Hotline
Box 1072
Hagerstown, Maryland
(301) 797-5050
Hotline refers for birth control, pregnancy tests, VD tests, abortion, and legal help. 7 P.M.–10 P.M. 7 days a week.

Hyattsville

Prince George's County Hotline for Youth
5611 Landover Rd.
Hyattsville, Maryland
(301) 864-7271
Hotline refers for birth control, pregnancy tests, VD tests, abortion, and legal help.

Rockville

Rockville Free Clinic
207 Maryland Ave.
Rockville, Maryland
(301) 424-3928
Free clinic offers birth control, pregnancy tests, VD tests, general medical care, and abortion referral. 24 hours, 7 days a week.

Seat Pleasant

Planned Parenthood of Prince George's County
5101 Pierce Ave., College Park
Seat Pleasant, Maryland
(301) 345-5252
Offers birth control and abortion referral.

Silver Spring

Somebody Cares
Colesville Rd. and Highland Drive
Silver Spring, Maryland
(301) 588-5440
Hotline and counseling service, refers for birth control, pregnancy tests, VD tests, and abortion. 8 P.M.–2 A.M. 7 days a week.

Towson

Brotherhood of Man
101 E. Joppa Rd.
Towson, Maryland
(301) 823-4357
Hotline and counseling service, refers for birth control, pregnancy tests, VD tests, abortion, and legal help.

Wheaton

Planned Parenthood of Montgomery County
1141 Georgia Ave., Room 420
Wheaton, Maryland
(301) 933-2300
Offers birth control, pregnancy tests, and abortion referral.

Montgomery County Hotline
Wheaton, Maryland
(301) 949-6603
Hotline refers for birth control, pregnancy tests, VD tests, abortion, and legal help. 24 hours, 7 days a week.

MASSACHUSETTS

Clergy Consultation Service on Abortion
(413) 586-3478
Statewide referral service for pregnancy tests and abortions.

Arlington

Arlington Youth Consultation Center
12 Prescott St.
Arlington, Massachusetts
(617) 643-1980
Hotline and counseling service, refers for birth control, pregnancy tests, VD tests, abortion, and legal help. 9 A.M.–11 P.M. 7 days a week.

Boston

Bridge Over Troubled Waters
Boston, Massachusetts
(617) 227-7114
Traveling medical van makes scheduled stops in Boston, Cambridge, and Chelsea 6:30 P.M.–midnight, Mon.–Fri. Offers pregnancy tests, VD tests, and general medical care. Call 10

A.M.–6 P.M. to find out stop in your area.

Dimock Community Health Center
Beth Israel Maternity and Infant Care Program
55 Dimock St.
Boston, Massachusetts
(617) 442-5700
Free clinic offers birth control, pregnancy tests, VD tests, and general medical care. 9 A.M.–5 P.M. Mon.–Fri.

Pregnancy Counseling Service
3 Joy St.
Boston, Massachusetts
(617) 523-1633, 1634
Offers pregnancy tests and abortion referral. 9 A.M.–5 P.M. Mon.–Fri.

Project Place
32 Rutland St.
Boston, Massachusetts
(617) 267-9150
Hotline and counseling service, refers for birth control, pregnancy tests, VD tests, abortion, and legal help. 24 hours, 7 days a week.

Brookline

Preterm
1842 Beacon St.
Brookline, Massachusetts
(617) 738-6210
Clinic offers birth control, pregnancy tests, VD tests, gynecological care, and abortion. $20 for first visit. 8 A.M.–6 P.M. Mon.–Fri.

Cambridge

Cambridgeport Free Clinic
10 Mt. Auburn St.
Cambridge, Massachusetts
(617) 876-0284
Free clinic offers birth control, pregnancy tests, VD tests, and general medical care. Recorded message tells you clinic hours.

Cambridgeport Problem Center
10 Mt. Auburn Street
Cambridge, Massachusetts
(617) 661-1010
Offers legal help and general counseling. 2 P.M.–5 P.M. Tues. and Thurs.

330 Evening Clinic for Young People
Mt. Auburn Hospital
330 Mt. Auburn St.
Cambridge, Massachusetts
(617) 492-3500, ext. 330
Clinic offers birth control, pregnancy tests, VD tests, general medical care, and abortion referral. Must call during the day to make an appointment. $12 for first visit.

Cambridge Hotline
595 Massachusetts Ave.
Cambridge, Massachusetts
(617) 876-7528
Hotline refers for birth control, pregnancy tests, VD tests, abortion, and legal help. 2 P.M.–2 A.M. 7 days a week.

Harvard Legal Aid Bureau
1511 Massachusetts Ave.
Cambridge, Massachusetts
(617) 495-4408
Hotline staffed by law students, offers legal help and information.

Lowell

Share/Morning Star

150 Middlesex St.
Lowell, Massachusetts
(617) 454-9981
Primarily a counseling service, also makes referrals for birth control, pregnancy tests, VD tests, and abortion. 9 A.M.–5 P.M. Mon.–Fri.

Lynn

Project Cope
117 N. Common St.
Lynn, Massachusetts
(617) 599-8020
Primarily a drug hotline, also makes referrals for birth control, pregnancy tests, VD tests, and abortion. 24 hours, 7 days a week.

Newton

Newton Hotline
Newton, Massachusetts
(617) 969-5906
Hotline and counseling service, refers for birth control, pregnancy tests, VD tests, abortion, and legal help. 8 P.M.–11 P.M. 7 days a week.

Planned Parenthood League of Massachusetts
93 Union St.
Newton Centre, Massachusetts
(617) 332-8750
Referral service for birth control, pregnancy tests, VD tests, and abortion.

Springfield

Springfield Hotline
Springfield College
Springfield, Massachusetts
(413) 781-7660
Hotline refers for birth control, pregnancy tests, VD tests, and abortion. 7 P.M.–11 P.M. 7 days a week.

Waltham

Waltham Helpline
Waltham, Massachusetts
(617) 891-4552
Hotline refers for birth control, pregnancy tests, VD tests, abortion, and legal help. 7 P.M.–midnight 7 days a week.

Watertown

Hotline, Helpline
463 Anarsenle St.
Watertown, Massachusetts
(617) 924-2210
Hotline and counseling service, refers for birth control, pregnancy tests, VD tests, abortion, and general medical care. 7 P.M.–midnight 7 days a week.

Worcester

Crisis Center
162 Chandler St.
Worcester, Massachusetts
(617) 791-6562
Hotline and counseling service, refers for birth control, pregnancy tests, VD tests, and abortion. 24 hours, 7 days a week.

MICHIGAN

Clergy Consultation Service on Abortion
(313) 964-0838
Statewide referral service for pregnancy tests and abortions.

Ann Arbor

Free People's Clinic
225 E. Liberty St.
Ann Arbor, Michigan
(313) 761-8952
Free clinic offers birth control, pregnancy tests, VD tests, general medical care, and abortion referral. Evenings. Mon.—Wed.

Express
912 N. Main
Ann Arbor, Michigan
(313) 662-1121
Planned Parenthood teen clinic, offers birth control, pregnancy tests, VD tests, and abortion referral.

Battle Creek

Help and Information Service
171 North Ave.
Battle Creek, Michigan
(616) 968-9276
Hotline and counseling service, refers for birth control, pregnancy tests, VD tests, and abortion. 10 A.M.–midnight Sun.–Thurs, 1 P.M.–1 A.M. Fri. and Sat.

Detroit

Project Headline
13627 Gratiot
Detroit, Michigan
(313) 526-5000
Free clinic and hotline, offers birth control, pregnancy tests, VD tests, general medical care, abortion referral, and general counseling. 24 hours, 7 days a week.

Y.E.S.
(Youth Education on Sex)
13100 Puritan
Detroit, Michigan
(313) 341-7708
Planned Parenthood teen clinic, offers birth control, pregnancy tests, VD tests, and abortion referral.

Flint

F.R.E.S.
(Flint Regional Emergency Service)
421 W. 5th Ave.
Flint, Michigan
(313) 235-5677
Hotline and counseling service, refers for birth control, pregnancy tests, VD tests, and abortion. 1 P.M.–1 A.M.

Flint Community Planned Parenthood Association
311 E. Court St.
Flint, Michigan
(313) 238-3631
Offers birth control, pregnancy tests, VD tests, and abortion referral. Special teen clinics.

Grand Rapids

Planned Parenthood Association of Kent County
425 Cherry, SE.
Grand Rapids, Michigan
(616) 459-3101
Offers birth control, pregnancy tests, VD tests, and abortion referral. Special teen clinics.

Switchboard
1330 Bradford NE
Grand Rapids, Michigan
(616) 456-3535
Hotline and counseling service, refers for birth control, pregnancy tests,

VD tests, abortion, and legal help. 24 hours, 7 days a week.

Kalamazoo

Gryphon Help Line
1104 S. Westnedge
Kalamazoo, Michigan
(616) 381-HELP
Hotline and counseling service, refers for birth control, pregnancy tests, VD tests, and abortion. 24 hours, 7 days a week.

Planned Parenthood Association of Kalamazoo County
612 Douglas Ave.
Kalamazoo, Michigan
(616) 349-8631
Offers birth control, pregnancy tests, VD tests, and abortion referral. Special teen clinic.

Lansing

Listening Ear
547 1/2 E. Grand River
Lansing, Michigan
(517) 337-1717
Hotline and counseling service, refers for birth control, pregnancy tests, VD tests, and abortion. 24 hours, 7 days a week.

Muskegon

Muskegon Area Planned Parenthood Association
1095 3rd St.
Muskegon, Michigan
(616) 722-2928
Offers birth control, pregnancy tests, and abortion referral.

MINNESOTA

Clergy Consultation Service on Abortion
(612) 545-8085
Statewide referral service for pregnancy tests and abortions.

Austin

Youth Emergency Service
2401 7th Ave. SW
Austin, Minnesota
(507) 437-6688
Hotline refers for birth control, pregnancy tests, VD tests, and abortion. 7 P.M.–1 A.M. 7 days a week.

Duluth

Planned Parenthood Clinic of St. Louis County
504 E. 2nd St.
Duluth, Minnesota
(218) 722-0833
Offers birth control, pregnancy tests, VD tests.

Mankato

Youth Emergency Service
1232 Highland Ave.
Mankato, Minnesota
(507) 387-4408
Hotline refers for birth control, pregnancy tests, VD tests, abortion, and legal help. 5 P.M.–1 A.M. 7 days a week.

Minneapolis

Youth Emergency Service

1429 Washington Ave. S.
(612) 339-7033
Hotline and counseling service, refers for birth control, pregnancy tests, VD tests, abortion, and legal help. 24 hours, 7 days a week.

Teenage Medical Service
2425 Chicago Ave. S.
Minneapolis, Minnesota
(612) 335-6408
Free clinic offers birth control, pregnancy tests, VD tests, gynecological care, and abortion referral. Recorded message will tell you clinic hours.

Beltrami Health Center
938 Lowry Ave. NE
Minneapolis, Minnesota
(612) 781-6816
Free clinic for residents of northeast Minneapolis, offers birth control, pregnancy tests, VD tests, gynecological care, and abortion referral.

Fremont Community Clinic
2507 Fremont Ave. N.
Minneapolis, Minnesota
(612) 529-9267
Free clinic for residents of north Minneapolis, offers birth control, pregnancy tests, VD tests, and gynecological care.

Planned Parenthood of Metropolitan Minneapolis
203 Walker Building
803 Hennepin Ave.
Minneapolis, Minnesota
(612) 336-8931
Offers birth control, pregnancy tests, VD tests, and abortion referral.

Northfield

Youth Emergency Service
402 S. Division St.
Northfield, Minnesota
(507) 645-4487
Hotline and counseling service, refers for birth control, pregnancy tests, VD tests, abortion, and legal help. 10 A.M.–midnight Mon.–Fri., 5 P.M.–midnight Sat. and Sun.

Rochester

Sunrise
119 1/2 1st Ave. NW
Rochester, Minnesota
(507) 288-0303
Hotline, refers for birth control, pregnancy tests, VD tests, abortion, and legal help. 9 A.M.–midnight 7 days a week.

Planned Parenthood of Minnesota, Southeast Region
116 1/2 S. Broadway
Rochester, Minnesota
(507) 288-5186
Offers birth control, pregnancy tests, and abortion referral.

St. Paul

Face to Face Crisis Center Clinic
716 Mendota St.
St. Paul, Minnesota
(612) 772-2557
Free clinic and counseling service, offers birth control, pregnancy tests, VD tests, gynecological care, and abortion referral. 9 A.M.–11 P.M. Mon.–Fri., 7 P.M.–2 A.M. Sat. and Sun.

Family Tree Clinic
1599 Selby Ave.
St. Paul, Minnesota
(612) 645-0478
Free clinic offers birth control, pregnancy tests, VD tests, and gynecological care. 9 A.M.–5 P.M. Mon.–Fri.

Planned Parenthood of Minnesota
Professional Plaza
1562 University Ave.
St. Paul, Minnesota
(612) 646-9603
Offers birth control, pregnancy tests, VD tests, and abortion referral.

Planned Parenthood of St. Paul Metropolitan Area
408 Hamm Building
408 St. Peter St.
St. Paul, Minnesota
(612) 224-1361
Offers birth control, pregnancy tests, VD tests, and abortion referral.

Winona

Youth Emergency Service
109 W. Broadway
Winona, Minnesota
(507) 452-5590
Hotline refers for birth control, pregnancy tests, VD tests, abortion, and legal help. 7 P.M.–3 AM. 7 days a week.

MISSISSIPPI

Clergy Consultation Service on Abortion
(601) 362-7075
Statewide referral service for pregnancy tests and abortions.

Biloxi

Help Line
PO Box 487
Biloxi, Mississippi
(601) 435-7200
(601) 374-4357
Hotline refers for birth control, pregnancy tests, VD tests, and abortion. 6 P.M.–midnight 7 days a week.

Jackson

Operation Venus
Gerow Hall
St. Josephs Hospital
Jackson, Mississippi
(601) 362-3939
VD hotline, offers information and referrals. 3 P.M.–5 P.M. Mon.–Fri.

Contact
PO Box 39211
Jackson, Mississippi
(601) 362-2525
Hotline refers for birth control, pregnancy tests, VD tests, and abortion. 24 hours, 7 days a week.

MISSOURI

Columbia

Everyday People
219 S. 6th St.
Columbia, Missouri
(314) 443-0424
Hotline and counseling service, refers for birth control, pregnancy tests, VD tests, abortion, and legal help. 24 hours, 7 days a week.

Planned Parenthood of Central Missouri

800 N. Providence Rd., Suite 5
Columbia, Missouri
(314) 443-0427
Offers birth control, pregnancy tests, and abortion referral.

Kansas City

Westport Free Clinic
4008 Baltimore
Kansas City, Missouri
(816) 931-3236
Free clinic offers birth control, VD tests, gynecological care, and general medical care. 10 A.M.–5 P.M. Mon.–Fri.

Planned Parenthood Association of Western Missouri/Kansas
4950 Cherry St.
Kansas City, Missouri
(816) 931-4121
Offers birth control, pregnancy tests, and abortion referral.

Human Rescue
PO Box 7624
Kansas City, Missouri
(816) 931-0030
Hotline refers for birth control, pregnancy tests, VD tests, abortion, and legal help. 24 hours, 7 days a week.

St. Louis

Family Planning Information Center
2202 S. Hanley
St. Louis, Missouri
(314) 647-2188
Referral service for birth control, pregnancy tests, VD tests, and abortion. 9 A.M.–5 P.M. Mon.–Fri.

Planned Parenthood Association of St. Louis
4947 Delmar Blvd.
St. Louis, Missouri
(314) 361-6360
Offers birth control, pregnancy tests, and abortion referral.

VD Information and Referral
1118 Hampton Ave.
St. Louis, Missouri
(314) 645-8355
VD hotline offers information and referrals. Also makes referrals for birth control and pregnancy tests. 9 A.M.–9 P.M. Mon.–Sat.

Youth Emergency Service
9307 Olive Rd.
St. Louis, Missouri
(314) 993-2292
Hotline refers for birth control, pregnancy tests, VD tests, and abortion. 24 hours, 7 days a week.

Springfield

Planned Parenthood of Southwest Missouri
1918 E. Meadowmere
Springfield, Missouri
(417) 869-6471
Offers birth control, pregnancy tests, VD tests, and abortion referral.

MONTANA

Billings

Crisis Center
PO Box 2519
Billings, Montana
(406) 245-6424
Hotline refers for birth control, pregnancy tests, VD tests, abortion, and legal help. 5 P.M.–7 A.M. 7 days a week.

Planned Parenthood of Billings

2718 Montana Ave.
Billings, Montana
(406) 252-2131
Offers birth control, pregnancy tests, VD tests, and abortion referral.

Missoula

Planned Parenthood of Missoula
Health Department Courthouse Annex
Room 213
Missoula, Montana
(406) 728-5490
Offers birth control, pregnancy tests, VD tests, and abortion referral.

NEBRASKA

Clergy Consultation Service on Abortion
(402) 453-5314
Statewide referral service for pregnancy tests and abortions.

Lincoln

Personal Crisis Service
Lincoln, Nebraska
(402) 475-5171
Hotline refers for birth control, pregnancy tests, VD tests, and abortion. 24 hours, 7 days a week.

Omaha

Equilibria
4924 Poppleton St.
Omaha, Nebraska
(402) 558-9977
Free clinic offers VD tests, gynecological care, and general medical care. 24 hours, 7 days a week.

Planned Parenthood of Omaha
2916 N. 58th St.
Omaha, Nebraska
(402) 554-1040
Offers birth control, pregnancy tests, and abortion referral.

Personal Crisis/Guideline
Omaha, Nebraska
(402) 342-6290
Hotline refers for birth control, pregnancy tests, VD tests, abortion, and legal help. 24 hours, 7 days a week.

NEVADA

Clergy Consultation Service on Abortion
(702) 565-4571
Statewide referral service for pregnancy tests and abortions.

Las Vegas

Operation Bridge Personal Crisis Hotline
116 Hoover St.
Las Vegas, Nevada
(702) 382-9690
Hotline and counseling service, refers for birth control, pregnancy tests, VD tests, abortion, and legal help. 24 hours, 7 days a week.

Planned Parenthood of Southern Nevada
1380 E. Sahara Ave.
Las Vegas, Nevada
(702) 734-9729
Offers birth control, pregnancy tests, and abortion referral.

Reno

Talk
Reno, Nevada
(702) 786-1119

Hotline refers for birth control, pregnancy tests, VD tests, and abortion. 3 P.M.—6 A.M. 7 days a week.

Crisis Center
Mack Social Science Building, Room 206
University of Nevada
Reno, Nevada
(702) 323-6111
Hotline and counseling service, refers for birth control, pregnancy tests, VD tests, and abortion. 24 hours, 7 days a week.

Planned Parenthood of Washoe County
505 N. Arlington
Reno, Nevada
(702) 323-8828
(702) 323-2159
Offers birth control, pregnancy tests, and abortion referral.

NEW HAMPSHIRE

Clergy Consultation Service on Abortion
(603) 646-2558
Statewide referral service for pregnancy tests and abortion.

Lebanon

Planned Parenthood Association of the Upper Valley
14 Parkhurst St.
Lebanon, New Hampshire
(603) 448-1214
Offers birth control, pregnancy tests, and abortion referral.

Manchester

Manchester Health Department
730 Elm St.
Manchester, New Hampshire
(603) 625-6428
Public health department offers VD tests and treatment, also refers for birth control, pregnancy tests, and abortion.

Family Planning
61 Amherst St.
Manchester, New Hampshire
(603) 669-7321
Birth-control clinic, also refers for pregnancy tests.

NEW JERSEY

Clergy Consultation Service on Abortion
(201) 933-2937
Statewide referral service for pregnancy tests and abortions.

Camden

Planned Parenthood, Greater Camden Area
590 Benson St.
Camden, New Jersey
(609) 365-3519
Offers birth control and abortion referral.

Glassboro

Together
7 State St.
Glassboro, New Jersey
(609) 881-4040
Hotline and counseling service, refers for birth control, pregnancy tests, VD tests, abortion, and legal help. 24 hours, 7 days a week.

Hackensack

Planned Parenthood of Bergen County
485 Main St.
Hackensack, New Jersey
(201) 489-1140
Offers birth control, pregnancy tests, and abortion referral.

Jersey City

Planned Parenthood Association of Hudson County
777 Bergen Ave. Room 218
Jersey City, New Jersey
(201) 332-2565
Offers birth control, pregnancy tests, and abortion referral.

Morristown

Planned Parenthood Center, Morris Area
197 Speedwell
Morristown, New Jersey
(201) 539-1364
Offers birth control, pregnancy tests, and abortion referral.

Newark

Planned Parenthood, Essex County
15 William St.
Newark, New Jersey
(201) 622-3900
Offers birth control and abortion referral.

Hotline
17 Mulberry St.
Newark, New Jersey
(201) 624-2405
Counseling service, also refers for birth control, pregnancy tests, VD tests, abortion, and legal help. 24 hours, 7 days a week.

New Brunswick

Planned Parenthood, Middlesex County
108 Bayard St.
New Brunswick, New Jersey
(201) 246-2404
Offers birth control, pregnancy tests, and abortion referral.

Paterson

Planned Parenthood of Passaic County
105 Presidential Blvd.
Paterson, New Jersey
(201) 274-4925
Offers birth control, pregnancy tests, VD tests, and abortion referral.

Plainfield

Planned Parenthood of Union County Area
234 Park Ave.
Plainfield, New Jersey
(201) 756-3736
Offers birth control, pregnancy tests, and abortion referral. Special teen clinics.

C.R.I. Hotline
232 E. Front St.
Plainfield, New Jersey
(201) 561-4800
Hotline refers for birth control, pregnancy tests, VD tests, and abortion. 7 P.M.–1 A.M. 7 days a week.

Princeton

Hotline

Princeton, New Jersey
(609) 924-1144
Hotline refers for birth control, pregnancy tests, VD tests, abortion, and legal help. 7 P.M.–midnight 7 days a week.

South Orange

S.O.S.
Seton Hall University
South Orange, New Jersey
(201) 762-1395
Hotline refers for birth control, pregnancy tests, VD tests, abortion, and legal help. 3 P.M.–midnight 7 days a week.

Trenton

Planned Parenthood of Mercer County
211 Academy St.
Trenton, New Jersey
(609) 599-4881
Offers birth control, pregnancy tests, VD tests, and abortion referral. Special teen clinics.

Health Department
City Hall
E. State St.
Trenton, New Jersey
(609) 392-3441, ext. 279 or ext. 280
Public health department offers VD tests and treatment.

Union

Communication Help Center
Newark State College
Morris Ave.
Union, New Jersey
(201) 527-2330
Hotline and counseling service, refers for birth control, pregnancy tests, VD tests, and abortion. 9 A.M.–1 P.M. Mon.–Fri., 2 P.M.–1 A.M. Sat. and Sun.

Wayne

Wayne Cares Hotline
50 Elmwood Terrace
Wayne, New Jersey
(201) 696-6019
Hotline refers for birth control, pregnancy tests, VD tests, abortion, and legal help. 24 hours, 7 days a week.

NEW MEXICO

Albuquerque

Youth Services Center
Bernalillo County Mental Health Center
2600 Marble NE
Albuquerque, New Mexico
(505) 265-3511, ext. 290
Counseling service, also refers for birth control, pregnancy tests, VD tests, abortion, and legal help. 9 A.M.–5 P.M. Mon.–Fri.

Four Corners Youth Services Center
122 Broadway SE
Albuquerque, New Mexico
(505) 843-6500
Drop-in center, also refers for birth control, pregnancy tests, VD tests, abortion, and legal help. 9 A.M.–9 P.M. Mon.–Fri.

Agora Student Crisis Center
Mesa Vista Building
University of New Mexico
Albuquerque, New Mexico

(505) 277-3013
Hotline and counseling service, refers for birth control, pregnancy tests, VD tests, abortion, and legal help. 9 A.M.–midnight 7 days a week.

Bernalillo County Planned Parenthood Association
113 Montclaire SE
Albuquerque, New Mexico
(505) 265-3722
Offers birth control, pregnancy tests, and abortion referral.

Fort Bayard

Planned Parenthood
Old Soldier Nurse Club
Fort Bayard, New Mexico
(505) 537-3093
Offers birth control and abortion referral.

Las Cruces

Planned Parenthood of Dona Ana County
221 W. Griggs Ave.
Las Cruces, New Mexico
(505) 524-8516
Offers birth control and abortion referral.

Santa Fe

Crisis Intervention
829 Allendale St.
Santa Fe, New Mexico
(505) 982-2771
Hotline refers for birth control, pregnancy tests, VD tests, and abortion. 24 hours, 7 days a week.

NEW YORK

Clergy Consultation Service on Abortion
(212) 254-6314
Statewide referral service for pregnancy tests and abortions.

Albany

Washington Park Free Medical Clinic
407 Hamilton St.
Albany, New York
(518) 463-4083
Free clinic offers pregnancy tests, VD tests, gynecological care, and general medical care. 6:30–9:30 P.M. Mon., Weds., Thurs.

Planned Parenthood Association of Albany
225 Lark St.
Albany, New York
(518) 434-2182
Offers birth control, pregnancy tests, and abortion referral. Special teen clinics.

Refer Switchboard
332 Hudson Ave.
Albany, New York
(518) 434-1202
Hotline refers for birth control, pregnancy tests, VD tests, abortion, and legal help. 24 hours, 7 days a week.

Binghamton

Planned Parenthoood of Broome County
710 O'Neil Building
Binghamton, New York
(607) 723-8306
Offers birth control, pregnancy tests, and abortion referral.

Buffalo

Planned Parenthood of Buffalo

210 Franklin St.
Buffalo, New York
(716) 853-1771
Offers birth control, pregnancy tests, and abortion referral.

Teens and Twenties Hotline
560 Main St.
Buffalo, New York
(716) 884-7900
Hotline and counseling service, refers for birth control, pregnancy tests, VD tests, abortion, and legal help. 4 P.M.–midnight 7 days a week.

East Meadow

Planned Parenthood of Nassau County
1940 Hempstead Turnpike
East Meadow, New York
(516) 292-8380
Offers birth control, pregnancy tests, and abortion referral.

Elmira

Planned Parenthood of the Southern Tier
200 E. Market St.
Elmira, New York
(607) 734-3313
Offers birth control, pregnancy tests, and abortion referral. Special teen clinics.

Huntington

Planned Parenthood Center of North Suffolk
17 E. Carver St.
Huntington, New York
(516) 427-7154
Offers birth control, pregnancy tests, and abortion referral. 9 A.M.–1 P.M. Mon.–Fri.

Ithaca

Open House
412 Linn St.
Ithaca, New York
(607) 273-1137
Hotline and counseling service, refers for birth control, pregnancy tests, VD tests, abortion, and legal help. 24 hours, 7 days a week.

Planned Parenthood of Tompkins County
512 E. State St.
Ithaca, New York
(607) 273-1513
Offers birth control, pregnancy tests, and abortion referral.

Mt. Vernon

Southern Westchester Planned Parenthood
16 S. 2nd Ave.
Mt. Vernon, New York
(914) 668-7927
Offers birth control, pregnancy tests, and abortion referral.

Newburgh

Planned Parenthood of Orange and Sullivan Counties
91 Dubois
Newburgh, New York
(914) 562-5748
Offers birth control, pregnancy tests, and abortion referral.

New York City

The Door
12 E. 12th St.
New York, New York
(212) 675-5405 medical clinic

(212) 675-9390 other services
Free clinic and counseling center, offers birth control, pregnancy tests, VD tests, gynecological care, abortion referral, and legal help. 6 P.M.–10 P.M. Mon.–Thurs.

Planned Parenthood of New York City
300 Park Ave. S.
New York, New York
(212) 777-2002
Referral service for birth control, pregnancy tests, VD tests, gynecological care, and abortion.

Planned Parenthood of New York City, 22nd St. Center
380 2nd Ave.
New York, New York
(212) 677-6474
Offers birth control, pregnancy tests, and abortion.

New York Switchboard
133 W. 4th St.
New York, New York
(212) 533-3186
Hotline refers for birth control, pregnancy tests, VD tests, abortion, and legal help. 10 A.M.–8 P.M. Mon.–Sat.

Lower West Side Public VD Clinic
303 9th Ave.
New York, New York
(212) 524-2537
Public health clinic offers VD tests and treatment.

Health Department VD Information
New York, New York
(212) 269-5300
Recorded message lists VD clinics in all five boroughs.

St. Mark's Free Clinic
44 St. Mark's Place
New York, New York
(212) 533-9500
Free clinic offers birth control, pregnancy tests, VD tests, and general medical care. 6 P.M.–10 P.M. Mon. and Weds.

Health Department Clearinghouse
New York, New York
(212) 233-3100
Public health department referral service for pregnancy tests and abortion.

Family Planning Information Service
New York, New York
(212) 677-3040
Referral service for birth control and abortion.

Niagara Falls

Planned Parenthood of Niagara County
906 Michigan
Niagara Falls, New York
(716) 282-1221
Offers birth control, pregnancy tests, and abortion referral.

Patchogue

Planned Parenthood of East Suffolk
119 N. Ocean Ave.
Patchogue, New York
(516) 475-5705
Offers birth control and abortion referral. 9 A.M.–1 P.M. Mon.–Fri.

Poughkeepsie

Planned Parenthood League of Dutchess County

85 Market St.
Poughkeepsie, New York
(914) 471-1540
Offers birth control, pregnancy tests, and abortion referral.

Rochester

The Center
293 Alexander St.
Rochester, New York
(716) 454-3083
Information center offers general counseling and legal help, also refers for birth control, pregnancy tests, VD tests, and abortion. 10 A.M.–11 P.M. Mon.–Sat.

Planned Parenthood League of Rochester and Monroe County
38 Windsor St.
Rochester, New York
(716) 546-2595
Offers birth control, pregnancy tests, and abortion referral.

Schenectady

Planned Parenthood League of Schenectady County
414 Union St.
Schenectady, New York
(518) 374-5353
Offers birth control, pregnancy tests, and abortion referral.

Syracuse

Ten Twelve
1305 E. Adams
Syracuse, New York
(315) 476-8370
(315) 476-DRUG
Free clinic and counseling center, offers birth control, pregnancy tests, VD tests, general medical care, and legal help. 24 hours, 7 days a week.

Planned Parenthood Center of Syracuse
1120 E. Genessee St.
Syracuse, New York
(315) 475-3193
Offers birth control, pregnancy tests, and abortion. Special teen clinics.

Utica

Planned Parenthood Association of the Mohawk Valley
11 Devereaux St.
Utica, New York
(315) 724-6146
Offers birth control, pregnancy tests, and abortion referral.

Watertown

Planned Parenthood of Northern New York, Jefferson County Chapter
161 Stone St.
Watertown, New York
(315) 788-8065
Offers birth control, pregnancy tests, and abortion referral.

West Nyack

Planned Parenthood of Rockland County
37 Village Square
West Nyack, New York
(914) 358-1145
Offers birth control, pregnancy tests, and abortion referral.

White Plains

Eastern Westchester Planned Parenthood Center

88 East Post Rd.
White Plains, New York
(914) 761-6566
(914) 948-5533 hotline
Offers birth control, pregnancy tests, and abortion referral. Hotline refers for these services throughout Westchester County.

Yonkers

Hudson River Planned Parenthood Center
45 Warburton Ave.
Yonkers, New York
(914) 965-1912
Offers birth control, pregnancy tests, and abortion referral.

NORTH CAROLINA

Clergy Consultation Service on Abortion
(919) 967-5333
Statewide referral service for pregnancy tests and abortions.

Charlotte

Planned Parenthood of Greater Charlotte
1416 E. Morehead St.
Charlotte, North Carolina
(704) 334-9563
Offers birth control, pregnancy tests, VD tests, and abortion referral.

Operation Venus
1200 Blythe Blvd.
Charlotte, North Carolina
(704) 374-2762
VD hotline offers information and referrals.

Durham

Edgemont Community Clinic
1012 E. Main St.
Durham, North Carolina
(919) 682-1750
Offers birth control, pregnancy tests, VD tests, general medical care, and abortion referral. 7 P.M.–11 P.M. Mon.–Thurs.

Greensboro

Switchboard
521 N. Edgeworth St.
Greensboro, North Carolina
(919) 275-0896
Hotline and counseling service, offers pregnancy tests and legal help, refers for birth control, VD tests, and abortion. 24 hours, 7 days a week.

Winston-Salem

Contact
1021-R Burke St.
Winston-Salem, North Carolina
(919) 722-5153
Hotline refers for birth control, pregnancy tests, VD tests, and abortion. 24 hours, 7 days a week.

NORTH DAKOTA

Bismarck

City Nursing Service
405 E. Broadway
Bismarck, North Dakota
(701) 223-9044
Public health clinic offers birth control, pregnancy tests, and VD tests.

Fargo

City Health Department of Fargo

City Hall
Fargo, North Dakota
(701) 235-7395
Public health clinic offers birth control, pregnancy tests, and VD tests.

OHIO

Clergy Consultation Service on Abortion
(216) 229-7423
Statewide referral service for pregnancy tests and abortions.

Akron

Ahead
633 E. Market St.
Akron, Ohio
(216) 535-5181
Free clinic and counseling service, offers pregnancy tests, VD tests, and general medical care. Also refers for birth control, abortion, and legal help. 24 hours, 7 days a week.

Planned Parenthood Association of Summit County
137 S. Main St.
Akron, Ohio
(216) 535-2671
Offers birth control, pregnancy tests, and abortion referral. Special teen clinics.

Canton

Planned Parenthood of Stark County
626 Walnut Ave. NE
Canton, Ohio
(216) 456-7191
Offers birth control, pregnancy tests, and abortion referral.

Cincinnati

Cincinnati Free Clinic
2444 Vine St.
Cincinnati, Ohio
(513) 621-5700
Free clinic offers birth control, pregnancy tests, VD tests, general medical care, and abortion referral. Noon–11 P.M. Mon.–Fri.

Planned Parenthood Association of Cincinnati
2406 Auburn Ave.
Cincinnati, Ohio
(513) 721-7635
Offers birth control, pregnancy tests, VD tests, and abortion referral.

Crisis Intervention Center
1620 Harrison Ave.
Cincinnati, Ohio
(513) 471-6000
(513) 471-HELP
Hotline and counseling center, refers for birth control, pregnancy tests, VD tests, abortion, and legal help. 9 A.M.–9 P.M. 7 days a week.

Cleveland

Free Medical Clinic of Greater Cleveland, Westside Branch
1985 W. 85th St.
Cleveland, Ohio
(216) 961-2323
Free clinic offers birth control, pregnancy tests, VD tests, general medical care, abortion referral, and general counseling.

Free Medical Clinic of Greater Cleveland, Eastside Branch
2039 Cornell Rd.
Cleveland, Ohio
(216) 721-4010
Free clinic offers birth control, preg-

nancy tests, VD tests, general medical care, abortion referral, and general counseling.

Planned Parenthood of Cleveland
2027 Cornell Rd.
Cleveland, Ohio
(216) 721-4700
Offers birth control, pregnancy tests, and abortion referral.

Columbus

Open Door Clinic
237 E. 17th Ave.
Columbus, Ohio
(614) 294-6337
Free clinic offers pregnancy tests, VD tests, and general medical care. Also refers for birth control and abortion. 10 A.M.–10 P.M.

Planned Parenthood Association of Columbus
206 E. State St.
Columbus, Ohio
(614) 224-8423
Offers birth control, pregnancy tests, and abortion referral.

Switchboard
118 King Ave.
Columbus, Ohio
(614) 294-6378
Hotline and counseling service, refers for birth control, pregnancy tests, VD tests, abortion, and legal help.

Dayton

Dayton Free Clinic and Counseling Center
10017 N. Main St.
Dayton, Ohio
(513) 288-2260
Free clinic offers birth control, pregnancy tests, VD tests, general medical care, abortion referral, general counseling, and legal help. 10 AM.–10 P.M.

Planned Parenthood Association of Miami Valley
224 North Wilkenson
Dayton, Ohio
(513) 226-0780
Offers birth control and abortion referral. Special teen clinics.

Mansfield

Planned Parenthood Association of the Mansfield Area
35 N. Park St.
Mansfield, Ohio
(419) 525-3075
Offers birth control, pregnancy tests, and abortion referral.

Newark

Planned Parenthood Association of East Central Ohio
17 N. 1st St.
Newark, Ohio
(614) 345-7445
Offers birth control, pregnancy tests, VD tests, and abortion referral.

Springfield

Planned Parenthood of West Central Ohio
401 N. Plum St.
Springfield, Ohio
(513) 325-7349
Offers birth control, pregnancy tests, and abortion referral.

Toledo

Planned Parenthood League of Toledo
217 15th St.

Toledo, Ohio
(419) 246-3651
Offers birth control, pregnancy tests, and abortion referral. Special teen clinics.

Rescue
4125 Monroe St.
Toledo, Ohio
(419) 473-2461
Hotline and counseling service, refers for birth control, pregnancy tests, VD tests, and abortion. 24 hours, 7 days a week.

Youngstown

Planned Parenthood of Mahoning Valley
125 W. Commerce St.
Youngstown, Ohio
(216) 746-5641
Offers birth control, pregnancy tests, and abortion referral.

OKLAHOMA

Oklahoma City

Paseo Clinic
133 NW 23rd
Oklahoma City, Oklahoma
(405) 524-8434
Free clinic offers birth control, pregnancy tests, VD tests, general medical care, and abortion referral. 7 P.M. Tues., Thurs., Sat.

Planned Parenthood Association of Oklahoma City
740 Culbertson Drive
Oklahoma City, Oklahoma
(405) 528-2157
Offers birth control, pregnancy tests, and abortion referral.

Youth Services for Oklahoma County
621 A NW 10th
Oklahoma City, Oklahoma
Referral service for birth control, pregnancy tests, VD tests, general medical care, abortion, and legal help.

Tulsa

Planned Parenthood Association of Tulsa
1615 E. 12th St.
Tulsa, Oklahoma
(918) 587-1101
Offers birth control, pregnancy tests, and abortion referral.

Hotline
Victorcrest Building
Tulsa, Oklahoma
(918) 583-4357
Hotline refers for birth control, pregnancy tests, VD tests, abortion, and legal help. 4 P.M.–1 A.M. 7 days a week.

OREGON

Eugene

Whitebird Socio-Medical Aid Station
341 E. 12th
Eugene, Oregon
(503) 342-8255
Free clinic offers pregnancy tests, VD tests, and general medical care. 24 hours, 7 days a week.

Planned Parenthood Association of Lane County
56 E. 15th St.
Eugene, Oregon
(503) 344-9411
Offers birth control, pregnancy tests, and abortion referral.

Medford

Planned Parenthood Association of Jackson County
650 Royal Ave., Suite 11
Medford, Oregon
(503) 773-8285
Referral service for birth control, pregnancy tests, VD tests, and abortion.

Portland

Outside-In
1236 SW Salmon
Portland, Oregon
(503) 223-4121
Free clinic and counseling service, offers pregnancy tests and general medical care. Also refers for birth control, VD tests, and abortion. 24 hours, 7 days a week.

Planned Parenthood Association
1200 SE Morrison
Portland, Oregon
(503) 234-5411
Offers birth control, pregnancy tests, and abortion referral.

Contact Center
Counseling and Resource Center
1532 SW Morrison
Portland, Oregon
(503) 226-4746
Hotline and counseling service, refers for birth control, pregnancy tests, VD tests, abortion, and legal help.

Community Action Program
1740 SE 139th
Portland, Oregon
(503) 252-0278
Hotline refers for birth control, pregnancy tests, VD tests, abortion, and legal help. 9 A.M.–5 P.M.

Portland Hotline
1740 SE 139th
Portland, Oregon
(503) 252-0278
Hotline refers for birth control, pregnancy tests, VD tests, abortion, and legal help. 6 P.M.–midnight.

Salem

Switchboard for Help/Cry of Love Clinic
1410 Fairgrounds Rd. NE
Salem, Oregon
(503) 581-5535
Hotline and free clinic, offers birth control, pregnancy tests, VD tests, general medical care, abortion referral, and legal help. 24 hours, 7 days a week.

PENNSYLVANIA

Clergy Consultation Service on Abortion
(215) 923-5141
Statewide referral service for pregnancy tests and abortions.

Operation Venus
(800) 462-4966
Statewide referral service for VD tests and treatment. Toll-free number.

Allentown

Planned Parenthood Association of Lehigh County
33 N. 5th St.
Allentown, Pennsylvania
(215) 439-1033
Referral service for birth control, pregnancy tests, VD tests, and abortion.

Easton

Planned Parenthood of Easton

415 Valley St.
Easton, Pennsylvania
(215) 252-3844
Offers birth control, pregnancy tests, and abortion referral.

Erie

Planned Parenthood Association of Erie County
G. Daniel Baldwin Building
1005 State St.
Erie, Pennsylvania
(814) 453-6473
Referral service for birth control, pregnancy tests, VD tests, and abortion.

Lancaster

Planned Parenthood of Lancaster
37 S. Lime St.
Lancaster, Pennsylvania
(717) 394-3575
Offers birth control, pregnancy tests, and abortion referral. Special teen clinics.

Philadelphia

Help
638 South St.
Philadelphia, Pennsylvania
(215) 928-0623
(215) 546-7766
Free clinic and counseling service, offers birth control, pregnancy tests, VD tests, general medical care, abortion referral, general counseling, and legal help. 24 hours, 7 days a week.

Operation Venus
213 Clover St.
Philadelphia, Pennsylvania
(215) LO 7-6969
(215) LO 7-6973
VD hotline, offers information about VD and will help arrange a confidential VD test.

Planned Parenthood Association of Southeastern Pennsylvania
1402 Spruce St.
Philadelphia, Pennsylvania
(215) 732-5880
Offers birth control, pregnancy tests, and abortion referral. Special teen clinics.

Public Health Department
Nursing Office
1440 Lombard St.
Philadelphia, Pennsylvania
(215) KI 6-0955, ext. 27
Public health referral service for pregnancy tests and VD tests.

Pittsburgh

Pittsburgh Free Clinic
East End Christian Church
S. Highland at Alder St.
Pittsburgh, Pennsylvania
(412) 661-5424
Free clinic offers birth control, pregnancy tests, VD tests, general medical care, and abortion referral.

Standby
PO Box 11262
Pittsburgh, Pennsylvania
(412) 782-4023
Hotline refers for birth control, pregnancy tests, VD tests, abortion, and legal help. 24 hours, 7 days a week.

Karma House
262 S. Bouquet St.
Pittsburgh, Pennsylvania
(412) 621-8555
Primarily for drug problems, also

refers for birth control, pregnancy tests, VD tests, and abortion.

Planned Parenthood Center of Pittsburgh
526 Penn Ave.
Pittsburgh, Pennsylvania
(412) 281-9502
Offers birth control, pregnancy tests, and abortion referral.

Reading

Planned Parenthood Center of Berks County
48 S. 4th St.
Reading, Pennsylvania
(215) 376-8061
Offers birth control, pregnancy tests, and abortion referral.

Scranton

Planned Parenthood Organization of Lackawanna County
316 N. Washington Ave.
Scranton, Pennsylvania
(717) 344-2626
Offers birth control, pregnancy tests, and abortion referral.

Wilkes-Barre

Planned Parenthood Association of Luzerne County
63 N. Franklin St.
Wilkes-Barre, Pennsylvania
(717) 824-8921
Offers birth control, pregnancy tests, and abortion referral.

Williamsport

Help Yourself
302 Locust St.
Williamsport, Pennsylvania
(717) 323-8444
Hotline refers for birth control, pregnancy tests, VD tests, abortion, and legal help. 24 hours, 7 days a week.

York

Planned Parenthood of York County
218 E. Market St.
York, Pennsylvania
(717) 845-9681
Offers birth control, pregnancy tests, and abortion referral.

RHODE ISLAND

Clergy Consultation Service on Abortion
(401) 331-7433
Statewide referral service for pregnancy tests and abortions.

Providence

Council of Community Services
Information Service
333 Grotto Ave.
Providence, Rhode Island
(401) 351-6500
Referral service for birth control, pregnancy tests, VD tests, general medical care, abortion, and legal help. 24 hours, 7 days a week.

Planned Parenthood of Rhode Island
46 Aborn St.
Providence, Rhode Island
(401) 421-9620
Offers birth control, pregnancy tests, and abortion referral. Special teen clinics.

SOUTH CAROLINA

Clergy Consultation Service on Abortion
(803) 268-1722

Statewide referral service for pregnancy tests and abortions.

Charleston

Public Health Department of Charleston County
334 Calhoun St.
Charleston, South Carolina
(803) 723-9251
Offers birth control, pregnancy tests, VD tests, and gynecological care. Also refers to neighborhood public health clinics.

Columbia

The Bosom Walk-In Center
709 Santee Ave.
Columbia, South Carolina
(803) 252-3601, walk-in center
(803) 758-2191, hotline
Hotline and counseling service, refers for birth control, pregnancy tests, VD tests, abortion, and legal help. 24 hours, 7 days a week.

Planned Parenthood of Central South Carolina
2014 Washington St.
Columbia, South Carolina
(803) 256-4908
Offers birth control and abortion referral.

Greenville

Crisis Intervention
Greenville, South Carolina
(803) 239-1021
Hotline refers for birth control, pregnancy tests, VD tests, and abortion.

SOUTH DAKOTA

Rapid City

Pennington County Health Department
615 Kansas City St.
Rapid City, South Dakota
(605) 342-0174
Public health clinic offers birth control, pregnancy tests, and VD tests.

Sioux Falls

City Health Department
City Hall
224 W. 9th St.
Sioux Falls, South Dakota
(605) 339-7075
Public health clinic offers birth control, pregnancy tests, VD tests, and gynecological care.

TENNESSEE

Clergy Consultation Service on Abortion
(615) 256-3441
Statewide referral service for pregnancy tests and abortions.

Chattanooga

Contact
1202 Duncan
Chattanooga, Tennessee
(615) 622-5193
Hotline refers for birth control, pregnancy tests, VD tests, abortion, and legal help. 24 hours, 7 days a week.

Knoxville

Planned Parenthood Association of

Knox County
114 Dameron Ave. NW
Knoxville, Tennessee
(615) 524-7487
Referral service for birth control, pregnancy tests, VD tests, and abortion.

Memphis

Runaway House
2117 Monroe
Memphis, Tennessee
(901) 276-1745
Counseling center and runaway house, refers for birth control, pregnancy tests, VD tests, abortion, and legal help. 24 hours, 7 days a week.

Memphis Planned Parenthood Association
9 N. 2nd St., Suite 1700
Memphis, Tennessee
(901) 525-0591
Offers birth control, pregnancy tests, and abortion referral.

Nashville

Rap House
1013 17th Ave. S.
Nashville, Tennessee
(615) 242-4281, hotline
(615) 255-7882, clinic
Free clinic and counseling service, offers birth control, pregnancy tests, VD tests, general medical care, and abortion referral. 24 hours, 7 days a week.

Planned Parenthood Center of Nashville
1114 17th Ave. S.
Nashville, Tennessee
(615) 255-7721
Offers birth control, pregnancy tests, and abortion.

Oak Ridge

Planned Parenthood Association of the Southern Mountains
162 Ridgeway Center
Oak Ridge, Tennessee
(616) 482-3406
Referral service for birth control, pregnancy tests, and abortion.

TEXAS

Clergy Consultation Service on Abortion
(214) 691-1282
Statewide referral service for pregnancy tests and abortions.

Amarillo

Panhandle Planned Parenthood Association
604 W. 8th
Amarillo, Texas
(806) 372-8731
Offers birth control, pregnancy tests, and abortion referral.

Austin

People's Free Clinic
408 W. 23rd St.
Austin, Texas
(512) 478-1746
Free clinic offers birth control, pregnancy tests, gynecological care, and general medical care. Mon.–Thurs.

Community Switchboard
2207 San Antonio St.

Austin, Texas
(512) 478-5657
Hotline and counseling service, refers for birth control, pregnancy tests, VD tests, abortion, and legal help. 3 P.M.–10 P.M.

Planned Parenthood Center of Austin
1823 E. 7th
Austin, Texas
(512) 477-5846
Offers birth control, pregnancy tests, and abortion referral.

Brownsville

Planned Parenthood of Cameron County
1158 E. Elizabeth St., Room 311
Brownsville, Texas
(512) 546-1048
Offers birth control and abortion referral.

Corpus Christi

Corpus Christi Drug Abuse Council
425 S. Broadway
Corpus Christi, Texas
(512) 883-7483
Crisis service primarily for drug problems. Also operates free clinic that offers pregnancy tests and VD tests. 24 hours, 7 days a week.

South Texas Planned Parenthood Center
622 Old Robstown Rd.
Corpus Christi, Texas
(512) 884-4352
Referral service for birth control, pregnancy tests, VD tests, and abortion.

Dallas

Planned Parenthood of Northeast Texas
3620 Maple Ave.
Dallas, Texas
(214) 521-3191
Offers birth control, pregnancy tests, and abortion referral.

El Paso

Planned Parenthood Center of El Paso
214 W. Franklin St.
El Paso, Texas
(915) 542-1919
Offers birth control and abortion referral.

Fort Worth

Our House
1417 8th Ave.
Fort Worth, Texas
(817) 923-9531
Hotline refers for birth control, pregnancy tests, VD tests, abortion, and legal help. 24 hours, 7 days a week.

Galveston

Crisis Hotline
Galveston, Texas
(713) 765-9416
Hotline and counseling service, refers for birth control, pregnancy tests, VD tests, abortion, and legal help. 24 hours, 7 days a week.

Houston

Crisis Hotline
Houston, Texas
(713) 228-1505
Hotline refers for birth control, pregnancy tests, VD tests, abortion, and legal help. 24 hours, 7 days a week.

Inlet Drug Crisis
704 Hawthorne
Houston, Texas
(713) 689-2196
Counseling service primarily for drug problems. Also refers for birth control, pregnancy tests, VD tests, and abortion. 1 P.M.–1 A.M. 7 days a week.

Planned Parenthood of Houston
3601 Fannin
Houston, Texas
(713) 522-3976
Offers birth control and abortion referral.

Lubbock

Planned Parenthood Association of Lubbock
3821 22nd St.
Lubbock, Texas
(806) 795-7123
Offers birth control, pregnancy tests, and abortion referral.

Odessa

Permian Basin Planned Parenthood
American Bank of Commerce Building, Suite 401
Odessa, Texas
(915) 563-2530
Offers birth control, pregnancy tests, VD tests, and abortion information.

San Antonio

San Antonio Free Clinic
1136 W. Woodlawn
San Antonio, Texas
(512) 732-4661
(512) 733-0383
Free clinic offers birth control, pregnancy tests, VD tests, general medical care, abortion referral, general counseling, and legal help. Noon–10 P.M. Mon.–Fri.

Planned Parenthood Center of San Antonio
106 Warren St.
San Antonio, Texas
(512) 227-2227
Offers birth control and abortion referral.

Waco

Planned Parenthood Center of Waco
1121 Ross Ave.
Waco, Texas
(817) 754-2307
Offers birth control, pregnancy tests, VD tests, and abortion referral.

Wichita Falls

Concern
Wichita Falls, Texas
(817) 723-0821
Hotline refers for birth control, pregnancy tests, VD tests, abortion, and legal help. 24 hours, 7 days a week.

UTAH

Provo

Crisis Line
1161 E. 300 North
Provo, Utah
(801) 375-5111
Hotline refers for birth control, pregnancy tests, VD tests, and abortion. 6 P.M.–midnight 7 days a week.

Salt Lake City

Planned Parenthood of Utah

1212 S. State St.
Salt Lake City, Utah
(801) 363-4471
Offers birth control and abortion counseling.

Listening Post
Salt Lake City, Utah
(801) 278-4716
Hotline refers for birth control, pregnancy tests, VD tests, abortion, and legal help. 24 hours, 7 days a week.

VERMONT

Barre

Barre Family Planning Center
24 Spaulding St.
Barre, Vermont
(802) 476-6696
Offers birth control, pregnancy tests, and problem-pregnancy information and referral.

Bennington

Bennington Family Planning Center
439 Main St.
Bennington, Vermont
(802) 442-3360
Offers birth control, pregnancy tests, and problem-pregnancy information and referral.

Brattleboro

Brattleboro Family Planning Center
21 Elliot St.
Brattleboro, Vermont
(802) 257-0102
Offers birth control, pregnancy tests, and problem-pregnancy information and referral.

Hotline/Fish
17 Elliot St.
Brattleboro, Vermont
(802) 257-7989
Hotline and counseling service, refers for birth control, pregnancy tests, VD tests, abortion, and legal help. 24 hours, 7 days a week.

Burlington

People's Free Clinic
260 North St.
Burlington, Vermont
(802) 864-6309
Free clinic offers birth control, pregnancy tests, VD tests, general medical care, and abortion referral.

Planned Parenthood Association of Vermont
19 Church St.
Burlington, Vermont
(802) 863-6326
Offers birth control, and problem-pregnancy information and referral. Special teen sessions.

The Place
260 College St.
Burlington, Vermont
(802) 658-3812
Hotline refers for birth control, pregnancy tests, VD tests, abortion, and legal help. 7:30 P.M.–midnight 7 days a week.

Vermont Women's Health Center
Exit 16 off Interstate 89
Colchester, Vermont
(802) 655-1600
Offers birth control, pregnancy tests, VD tests, gynecological care, and abortion. 9 A.M.–4 P.M. Tues.–Sat.

Rutland

Rutland Family Planning Center
46 1/2 Center St.
Rutland, Vermont
(802) 775-2333
Offers birth control, pregnancy tests, and problem-pregnancy information and referral.

VIRGINIA

Clergy Consultation Service on Abortion
(703) 951-2516
Statewide referral service for pregnancy tests and abortions.

Alexandria

Alexandria Hotline
101 N. Columbus St.
Alexandria, Virginia
(703) 548-3810
Hotline refers for birth control, pregnancy tests, VD tests, abortion, and legal help. 24 hours, 7 days a week.

Arlington

Northern Virginia Hotline
Arlington, Virginia
(703) 527-4077
Hotline refers for birth control, pregnancy tests, VD tests, abortion, and legal help. 24 hours, 7 days a week.

Charlottesville

Planned Parenthood of Central Virginia
1106 W. Main St., Room 3
Charlottesville, Virginia
(804) 296-1777
Referral service for birth control, pregnancy tests, VD tests, and abortion.

Falls Church

Planned Parenthood of Northern Virginia
5827 Columbia Pike
Falls Church, Virginia
(703) 820-3335
Offers birth control, pregnancy tests, and abortion referral.

Hampton

Peninsula Planned Parenthood
92 LaSalle Ave.
Hampton, Virginia
(804) 826-2079
Referral service for birth control, pregnancy tests, VD tests, and abortion. 9 A.M.–1 P.M. Mon.–Fri.

Lynchburg

Greater Lynchburg Planned Parenthood
1503 Grace St.
Lynchburg, Virginia
(804) 846-6093
Referral service for birth control, pregnancy tests, VD tests, and abortion.

Newport News

Contact
211 32nd St.
Newport News, Virginia
(804) 245-0041
Referral service for birth control, pregnancy tests, VD tests, abortion, and legal help. 24 hours, 7 days a week.

Norfolk

Norfolk Free Clinic
535 Boissevain Ave.
Norfolk, Virginia
(804) 625-5444
Free clinic offers birth control, pregnancy tests, VD tests, general medical care, abortion referral, and general counseling. 7 P.M.—10 P.M. Mon.—Fri.

Information Center of Hampton Rose
500 E. Plume
Norfolk, Virginia
(804) 625-4543
Hotline refers for birth control, pregnancy tests, VD tests, abortion, and legal help. 9 A.M.–5 P.M. Mon.–Fri.

Planned Parenthood of Norfolk
Norfolk Public Health Center
401 Colley Ave., Room 113
Norfolk, Virginia
(804) 625-5591
Referral service for birth control, pregnancy tests, VD tests, and abortion.

Richmond

Fan Free Clinic
1721 Hanover Ave.
Richmond, Virginia
(804) 358-8538
Free clinic offers birth control, pregnancy tests, VD tests, and general medical care. 10 A.M.–1 P.M. Mon.—Fri.,EveningsTues.andThurs.

Youth Emergency Service
Richmond, Virginia
(804) 355-3256
Hotline refers for birth control, pregnancy tests, VD tests, abortion, and legal help. 4 P.M.–10 P.M. Mon.–Thurs., 6 P.M.–midnight Fri.–Sun.

Virginia League for Planned Parenthood
2009 Monument Ave.
Richmond, Virginia
(804) 358-4919
Referral service for birth control, pregnancy tests, VD tests, and abortion.

Roanoke

Trust
3515 Williamson Rd.
Roanoke, Virginia
(703) 563-0311
Hotline and counseling service, refers for birth control, pregnancy tests, VD tests, and legal help. Also does problem-pregnancy counseling. 24 hours, 7 days a week.

Roanoke Valley League for Planned Parenthood
920 S. Jefferson St.
Roanoke, Virginia
(703) 342-6741
Referral service for birth control, pregnancy tests, VD tests, and abortion.

Virginia Beach

Virginia Beach Planned Parenthood
107 45th St.
Virginia Beach, Virginia
(804) 425-1908
Referral service for birth control, pregnancy tests, VD tests, and abortion. 10 A.M.–2 P.M. Mon.–Fri.

WASHINGTON

Bellingham

The Rising Sun
1020 N. Forest
Bellingham, Washington
(206) 733-9212
Crisis intervention center, also refers for birth control, pregnancy tests, VD tests, and abortion.

Planned Parenthood of Whatcom County
220 W. Champion St., Room 200
Bellingham, Washington
(206) 734-9095
Offers birth control, pregnancy tests, and abortion referral.

Everett

Planned Parenthood of Snohomish County
1508 Hewitt Ave.
Everett, Washington
(206) 259-0096
Offers birth control, pregnancy tests, and abortion referral.

Olympia

Crisis Clinic
Evergreen State College
Olympia, Washington
(206) 357-3681
(206) 357-3683
Hotline refers for birth control, pregnancy tests, VD tests, abortion, and legal help. 24 hours, 7 days a week.

Seattle

Planned Parenthood Center of Seattle
202 16th Ave. S.
Seattle, Washington
(206) 329-3625
Offers birth control, pregnancy tests, and abortion referral.

Open Door Free Clinic
5012 Roosevelt Way NE
Seattle, Washington
(206) 524-7404
Free clinic and hot line, offers birth control, pregnancy tests, VD tests, general medical care, and general counseling. 24 hours, 7 days a week.

Aradia Women's Clinic
4224 University Way NE
Seattle, Washington
(206) 634-2090
Offers birth control, pregnancy tests, VD tests, gynecological care, and abortion referral. Mon. and Thurs. evening, Tues. and Weds. afternoons.

County Doctor Clinic
402 15th Ave. E.
Seattle, Washington
(206) 322-6698
Offers birth control, pregnancy tests, VD tests, general medical care, and abortion referral.

The Brotherhood
9067 53rd Ave. S.
Seattle, Washington
(206) 723-1881
Hotline refers for birth control, pregnancy tests, VD tests, abortion, and legal help. 24 hours, 7 days a week.

Crisis Clinic
1701 17th

Seattle, Washington
(206) 323-2100, information service
(206) 329-3201, teenage hotline
Hotline refers for birth control, pregnancy tests, VD tests, and abortion.

Spokane

Planned Parenthood of Spokane
E. 2202 Sprague
Spokane, Washington
(509) 535-9747
Referral service for birth control, pregnancy tests, VD tests, and abortion.

Tacoma

Planned Parenthood of Pierce County
4002 S. M St.
Tacoma, Washington
(206) 475-5123
Offers birth control, pregnancy tests, and abortion referral.

Crisis Clinic
Tacoma, Washington
(206) 383-2042, main number
(206) 383-1661, teenage hotline
Hotline refers for birth control, pregnancy tests, VD tests, abortion, and legal help.

Walla Walla

Center for Family Planning
329 S. 2nd St.
Walla Walla, Washington
(509) 529-3570
Offers birth control, pregnancy tests, and abortion referral.

Yakima

Planned Parenthood Association of Yakima County
208 N. 3rd Ave.
Yakima, Washington
(509) 248-3625
Offers birth control, pregnancy tests, and abortion referrals.

WEST VIRGINIA

Charleston

County Health Department
Nursing Office
PO Box 927
Charleston, West Virginia
(304) 348- 8150
Health department refers to neighborhood clinics for birth control, pregnancy tests, VD tests, and gynecological care.

Huntington

Contact
Huntington, West Virginia
(304) 523-3448
Hotline refers for birth control, pregnancy tests, VD tests, and abortion. 24 hours, 7 days a week.

WISCONSIN

Clergy Consultation Service on Abortion
(414) 352-4050
Statewide referral service for pregnancy tests and abortions.

Eau Claire

Tap Line
310 Chestnut
Eau Claire, Wisconisn
(715) 834-1212
Hotline refers for birth control, preg-

nancy tests, VD tests, abortion, and legal help. 24 hours, 7 days a week.

Green Bay

Planned Parenthood of Green Bay
130 E. Walnut St., Suite 501
Green Bay, Wisconsin
(414) 432-0031
Offers birth control and abortion referral.

Kenosha

Planned Parenthood of Kenosha
Kenosha, Wisconsin
(414) 657-6211
Offers birth control, pregnancy tests, VD tests, and abortion referral.

Madison

Rap Center
923 Spring St.
Madison, Wisconsin
(608) 257-3522
Hotline and counseling service, refers for birth control, pregnancy tests, VD tests, abortion, and legal help. 8 P.M.—midnight Mon.—Sat.

Blue Bus Free Clinic
222 N. Bassett
Madison, Wisconsin
(608) 262-7330
(608) 262-5889
Free clinic offers pregnancy tests, VD tests, and general medical care. Also refers for birth control and abortion. 7 P.M.–9:30 P.M. Mon., Weds., Fri.

Milwaukee

Planned Parenthood Association of Wisconsin
1135 W. State St.
Milwaukee, Wisconsin
(414) 271-8181
Offers birth control and pregnancy tests.

Problem Pregnancy Information Service
2266 N. Prospect Ave.
Milwaukee, Wisconsin
(414) 276-6207
Offers abortion referral and counseling.

Survival Center
929 E. Pearson
Milwaukee, Wisconsin
(414) 272-3409
Hotline and counseling service, refers for birth control, pregnancy tests, VD tests, abortion, and legal help. 24 hours, 7 days a week.

Underground Switchboard
St. Mary's Hospital
2390 North Lake Drive
Milwaukee, Wisconsin
(414) 271-3123, hotline
(414) 271-8423, clinic
Hotline and free clinic, offers VD tests and general medical care. Also refers for birth control, pregnancy tests, and abortion. 2 P.M.–2 A.M. 7 days a week.

WYOMING

Cheyenne

Helpline
Cheyenne, Wyoming
(307) 634-4469
Hotline refers for birth control, pregnancy tests, VD tests, abortion,

and legal help. 6 P.M.–11 P.M. 7 days a week.

Laramie

Laramie Cares
Laramie, Wyoming
(307) 742-3793
Hotline refers for birth control, pregnancy tests, VD tests, abortion, and legal help. 9 A.M.–midnight.

NATIONAL SERVICES

Clergy Consultation Service on Abortion
(212) 254-6314
Referral service for pregnancy tests and abortions. If there is no Clergy Consultation Service chapter listed under your state, this New York office can give you the name of the counselor in your area.

Family Planning Information Service
(212) 677-3040
Nationwide abortion referral service operated by Planned Parenthood. Make sure your pregnancy test is positive before calling this service.

Operation Venus
(800) 523-1885
Nationwide VD referral service. Counselors at this toll-free number can give you information about VD and tell you where to get a VD test in any part of the country.

Dictionary

ANUS: the tight ring of muscle at the opening of the rectum—the asshole.

BISEXUAL: any person, either a man or a woman, who likes to have sex with both males and females.

CERVIX: the neck of the uterus, which hangs down into the vagina. The tiny hole in the cervix connects a woman's vagina with the rest of her internal reproductive organs.

CONTRACEPTION: any kind of birth control that prevents a man's sperm from fertilizing a woman's egg and therefore prevents a pregnancy.

CUNNILINGUS: the technical term for stimulating a woman's genitals with your mouth.

DOUCHE: rinsing out the inside of the vagina. It's usually done with a special rubber bag and nozzle that allows water to flow in and out of the vagina.

EJACULATION: the squirting of semen from a man's penis that happens at orgasm.

EMANCIPATION: a legal term that means a minor is no longer under the care or control of his parents. In most states you have to be at least sixteen, self-supporting, and living on your own in order to be considered emancipated.

EROGENOUS ZONES: those areas of the body that are highly sensitive to sexual stimulation, including the genitals, the breasts, the buttocks, the thighs, and the whole area around the sex organs.

ESTROGEN: a female sex hormone produced by a woman's ovaries. Synthetic estrogen is one of the two hormones in birth-control pills.

FALLOPIAN TUBES: the two small tubes that connect a woman's ovaries with her uterus. Eggs pass through the fallopian tubes on their way from the ovaries to the uterus.

FELLATIO: the technical term for stimulating a man's penis with your mouth.

FERTILE: capable of having children. A man is fertile when his testicles are producing healthy sperm. A woman is fertile when her ovaries are releasing ripe eggs.

FERTILIZATION: the beginning of a pregnancy, it happens when a sperm cell penetrates an egg.

GENITALS: the external sex organs. A man's genitals are the penis and the testicles. A woman's genitals are the vagina, the vaginal lips, and the clitoris.

GYNECOLOGY: a branch of medicine that deals with a woman's sex organs and reproductive system.

HETEROSEXUAL: a person who is sexually oriented toward the opposite sex. In other words, a man who is attracted to women or a woman who is attracted to men.

HOMOSEXUAL: a person who is sexually oriented toward his own sex. That is, a man who is attracted to other men or a woman who is attracted to other women.

HORMONE: a chemical substance produced by your body that affects the way your body functions. A man's sex hormones are produced by his testicles, a woman's sex hormones are produced by her ovaries.

HYMEN: a thin membrane that blocks the entrance to the vagina.

IMPOTENCE: not being able to get an erection. Impotence is something that happens to almost all men at one time or another when they can't get an erection because of nervousness, fatigue, drugs, etc. If it happens all the time, then it's a serious problem that needs medical attention.

INTERCOURSE: insertion of the penis into the vagina.

LABIA MAJORA: the technical name for the outer lips of the vagina.

LABIA MINORA: the technical name for the inner lips of the vagina.

LESBIAN: a female homosexual, a woman whose primary sexual interest is other women.

MENSTRUAL CYCLE: the series of changes that take place in a woman's body from one menstrual period to the next. The menstrual cycle is measured from the first day of a woman's period, and during each cycle the uterus sheds its lining, the ovaries produce a ripe egg, and the uterus builds a new lining. The menstrual cycle is controlled by the flow of sex hormones in a woman's body.

ORGASM: the physical release of sexual tension that happens when a person reaches maximum sexual excitement. A man's orgasm is accompanied by ejaculation of semen from the penis. A woman's orgasm is accompanied by contractions inside the vagina.

OVARIES: the two female sex glands that produce eggs and female hormones.

OVULATION: the process that takes place once during each menstrual cycle when a woman's ovaries release a ripe egg.

PROGESTERONE: a female sex hormone produced by the ovaries. Synthetic progesterone is one of the two hormones used in birth-control pills.

PROPHYLACTIC: a condom or rubber.

PROSTATE GLAND: the gland that produces part of the liquid that goes into a man's semen. The prostate gland is located below a man's bladder and touches the wall of his rectum.

PUBERTY: the period during which your body first develops adult sexual characteristics and becomes capable of having children.

RECTUM: the end of the large intestines up inside the anus.

REPRODUCTION: the technical term for having children.

REPRODUCTIVE ORGANS: the sex organs of both men and women that are responsible for pregnancy and childbirth.

SCROTUM: the crinkly sack of skin below a man's penis that holds his testicles.

SEMEN: the fluid that is ejaculated from a man's penis. Semen is made up of sperm plus liquids that are secreted from several glands inside a man's body.

SEMINAL VESICLES: two tiny reservoirs inside a man's body that store sperm until it is ejaculated. The seminal vesicles also produce some of the liquid that makes up semen.

SODOMY: a legal and religious term for inserting the penis into the mouth or anus. The word is chiefly used to describe the sexual activity of male homosexuals.

SPERMICIDE: a chemical that kills sperm.

STERILE: unable to have children. A man is sterile if his testicles don't produce healthy sperm. A woman is sterile if her ovaries don't produce ripe eggs.

SUPPOSITORY: a medicated tablet that melts when it's inserted into the vagina or anus.

TESTICLES: the male sex glands that produce sperm and male sex hormones. They hang in a sack of skin below the penis.

TESTOSTERONE: a male sex hormone produced by the testicles.

URETHRA: the tube that carries urine from the bladder to the outside world. In men the opening to the urethra is located in the tip of the penis. In women the opening to the urethra is located between the vagina and the clitoris.

UTERUS: the pear-shaped organ inside a woman's abdomen that's designed to hold and feed an unborn child. When a woman is not pregnant, the lining of the uterus is shed each month during menstruation.

VULVA: a woman's external sex organs, including the outer lips, the inner lips, the clitoris, the urethral opening, and the entrance to the vagina.